Dear Harriet & Joel,

Good friends, as
rare wines, just get
better as they age.
And so it is with
us.

Love you both
very much!

Hugs & more,

Lois

Sex, Lies and Cosmetic Surgery

Things You'll Never Learn From Your Plastic Surgeon

by

Lois W. Stern

Foreword by David B. Sarwer Ph.D.

ISBN 0-7414-3220-X

Published by:

INFI∞ITY
PUBLISHING.COM

1094 New DeHaven Street, Suite 100
West Conshohocken, PA 19428-2713
Info@buybooksontheweb.com
www.buybooksontheweb.com
Toll-free (877) BUY BOOK
Local Phone (610) 941-9999
Fax (610) 941-9959

Printed in the United States of America

Printed on Recycled Paper

Published September 2006

Acknowledgements

My heartfelt gratitude and sincere words of thanks go to the following people:

My husband, Ken, who has always been there for me
> There would be no book without your patience, understanding and support.

The many women who contributed to *Sex, Lies and Cosmetic Surgery,* by sharing their personal experiences and thoughtful insights
> The depth and candor of your contributions have enriched the contents of this book immeasurably.

The plastic surgeons, nurses, anesthesiologists, psychologists, estheticians and others who work with cosmetic surgery patients daily
> Your willingness to share your individual areas of expertise, born of years of experience in your specific disciplines, has enabled me to now reach out to enrich others.

Dr. David B. Sarwer, Associate Professor of Psychology and Psychiatry at the University of Pennsylvania School of Medicine, who gently but steadfastly guided me in my pursuit of the research for *Sex, Lies and Cosmetic Surgery*
> You have helped me validate much of the anecdotal contents of my book through your able guidance. Your support has been invaluable.

Denise Thomas, Manhattan's Cosmetic Surgery Consultant, for her enthusiasm, thoughtful input and perceptive insights
> You have given generously both of your time and your many contacts to help give shape to the anecdotal, human interest stories within this book.

My editor, Joanne Starer, for her unflinching objectivity,
savvy advice and immutable magic touch
It was a pleasure to work with you throughout the process of
refining my manuscript. You turned what could have been
drudgery into an exciting new challenge.

Linda Langton, of Langtons International
Your early belief in this project helped energize me.
Thank you for your encouragement and guidance.

The terrific team at Infinity Publishing, including:
John Harnish, Special Projects Director, for his
helpful advice and the many courtesies he has
extended to me
Michelle Shane, for her attentive responses to my many
questions
Chris Master, for his attention to fine detail while
creating the cover for *Sex, Lies
and Cosmetic Surgery*.

And finally, my many friends who encouraged me during
these past five years
By tolerating my absences and obsessive focus on my work,
you have lent your unspoken support.

Table of Contents

Page

Foreword *1*

Introduction **v**

**Chapter 1: Cosmetic Surgery –
The Aphrodisiac Effect** **1**
- The strong sexual overtones to cosmetic surgery
- The lifetime link between physical appearance, sexuality and sexual opportunities
- Women's intimate experiences

Chapter 2: Sexuality on the Home Front **19**
- My upfront and personal story following cosmetic surgery

Chapter 3: What to Expect After Cosmetic Surgery **25**
- Altered self-perceptions, emotions, relationships
- Long range health and longevity studies of women who have undergone cosmetic surgery
- Possible health related benefits to looking good

Chapter 4: Preferential Treatment For the Pretty Ones **41**
- Attraction to beauty begins nearly at birth
- How the physical attractiveness stereotype is perpetuated amongst adults
- Women's post surgery experiences with friends, spouses, partners, family members, and casual acquaintances
- When beauty is only skin deep
- Limitations to the physical attractiveness stereotype

Chapter 5: Utter Humiliation   55

- Embarrassing moments - Unexpected feelings toward my surgeon
- Six tips for cosmetic surgery patients
- Six tips for plastic surgeons

Chapter 6: You Might Fall in Love with Your Plastic Surgeon   69

- Women speak of their personal experiences with this not uncommon phenomenon
- Professionals speak out

Chapter 7: What Propels Us   81

- Motivations and catalysts to the decision to undergo cosmetic surgery
- Women's secret and hidden motivations

Chapter 8: What Deters Us   103

- Underlying ambivalent feelings
- In-depth interviews with five women who said "no" to cosmetic surgery and why
- Sorting through your personal ambivalences

Chapter 9: Secrecy, Deception and Lies   121

- Evolving attitudes about privacy, secrecy and candor following cosmetic surgery
- Why many women opt for less than full disclosure
- Some inventive deceptions and convincing scripts for those who want to guard their secret
- You may be happier afterwards, but don't expect everyone to share your happiness.

Chapter 10: Misperceptions and Misconceptions   145
- Faulty insights and misunderstandings surrounding plastic surgery
- That unfortunate wind tunnel look for those subjected to poor quality facelifts
- Words of wisdom from women who have experienced post surgical setbacks

Chapter 11: Changing Attitudes: From Freud to the 21st Century   169
- Evolving attitudes toward cosmetic surgery: Psychopathological theories give way to theories of normalcy
- The current explosion in cosmetic surgery numbers
- Have we gone too far?
- The 'typical' woman who goes for cosmetic surgery today
- Body Dysmorphic Disorder (BDD) - How this syndrome fits into the cosmetic surgery equation

Chapter 12: Time for a Bit of Satire – Step Right Then Step Left   187
- Fictional accounts of two worlds with opposite-to-the-extreme views about the importance of beauty
- Our society's growing trend toward earlier and more cosmetic surgery
- Updated statistics, media madness and other forms of hype

Chapter 13: Brain Sex, Women and   **199**
    Cosmetic Surgery
- A concluding joke to highlight ways men and women typically think and respond differently, both emotionally and sexually
- What causes male and female brains to function differently?
  - Do gender specific brain differences relate to women's attraction to cosmetic surgery?
  - Do gender specific brain differences impact women's sexuality after cosmetic surgery?

Epilogue   **217**

I wrote this epilogue to respond to the questions most often posed to me:

- How did I find my plastic surgeon?
- What was the day of surgery really like?
- Did I experience much pain?
- How did I feel with my first post surgery look in the mirror?
- How long did it take to heal?

I answer these questions and more as I share both my experiences and a serendipitous moment several months post surgery that reaffirmed my conviction that I had chosen well.

Afterwords   **254**

I offer a few words of advice about healthy living after surgery and conclude with the basic foundation of this book: Be honest and true to yourself. If you have reason to consider your views well founded, stand by them. I do and I have, as have the over one hundred people who contributed to this book.

Page

Forms, Checklists and Quizzes   **261**

Appendices   **300**

CD Order Form   **383**

About the Author   **385**

Foreword

According to the American Society of Plastic Surgeons, over 11.5 million Americans underwent a cosmetic surgical or minimally invasive procedure in 2005. This statistic, while familiar to plastic surgeons, is often staggering to those who have little idea of the number of Americans who turn to plastic surgery to enhance their physical appearance. In reality, 11.5 million is likely an underestimate of the number of persons who undergo cosmetic surgery each year, as this figure does not account for the increasing number of medical professionals who now offer these treatments. Regardless, the sheer number of individuals who undergo these procedures reflects society's increased acceptance of improving one's appearance by medical means.

Several factors have likely contributed to the tremendous growth in popularity of cosmetic surgery over the past decade. Changes in the medical and surgical communities, including improvements in safety and the proliferation of direct-to-consumer marketing, likely have increased the demand for cosmetic surgery. The mass media has long championed cosmetic surgery, perhaps no more so than during the current era of widely watched "reality-based" television programs such as "Extreme Makeover", "The Swan", and "Dr. 90210". These shows are just a small part of a virtually inescapable bombardment of mass media ideals of beauty from magazines, television shows, movies and the Internet that we are exposed to on a daily basis.

Without question, exposure to these images contributes to our collective dissatisfaction with our physical appearance. More than half of American women and slightly less than half of American men report being dissatisfied with their appearance. To address this dissatisfaction, we spend tens of billions of dollars each year on weight loss products, health club memberships, cosmetics purchases, and, increasingly, on cosmetic surgery.

As if these factors weren't enough, numerous studies over the past several decades have found that not only are attractive people judged more favorably by others, but that they also receive preferential treatment in a range of interpersonal interactions across the life span. Simply put, whether we like to admit it or not, our appearance seems to matter. Considering all of these influences together, the interest in and growth of cosmetic surgery is not particularly surprising.

In Lois Stern's **Sex, Lies, and Cosmetic Surgery**, we are reminded that, even if we consider all of these factors, the decision to seek cosmetic surgery is quite individualized. From her detailed account of her own experience with surgery, to her interviews with other women who have undergone surgery, Stern shares with us the many stories that lead to and from the plastic surgeon's office. Plastic surgeons and mental health professionals have long been interested in the psychological characteristics of cosmetic surgery patients. Decades ago, a person's interest in cosmetic surgery was often dismissed as trivial vanity or unbridled narcissism. Today, we are more likely to see an individual's pursuit of surgery as a positive self-care strategy--analogous to eating a healthy diet or exercising regularly--than we are to see it as a symptom of a significant psychological problem.

As described in the book and supported by the research, improving one's appearance and body image—the internal representation of one's external appearance—is believed to be a central motivation for many cosmetic surgery patients. Body image is considered to be an important element of one's self esteem and quality of life. In turn, sexuality—one of the major themes of *Sex, Lies, and Cosmetic Surgery*--is an important aspect of body image for many individuals.

Given the relationships between sexuality, body image, and cosmetic surgery, it is not surprising that some women report becoming sexually or romantically attracted to their surgeon. We can become attracted to those who, in the course of social and professional interaction, become physically close to us and make us feel good about ourselves. These experiences of interpersonal warmth and intimacy often lead to sexual attraction. Stern does readers a great favor in examining this "don't ask, don't tell" experience and underscoring the need to keep appropriate professional boundaries between physician and patient.

Perhaps the greatest value of *Sex, Lies, and Cosmetic Surgery* lies in the breadth of stories found within its pages. Until recently, cosmetic surgery was thought to be reserved only for a certain, select subset of women. Today, an increasing number of women (and men) from a range of age, socioeconomic and ethnic groups undergo cosmetic surgery. There is no doubt that there are commonalities between these women, yet there also are countless individual differences. How and when did she become dissatisfied with her appearance? How did she find a surgeon with whom she felt comfortable? How scared was she? How much did it hurt? Who did she tell? How did she look and feel afterwards? All of these questions, and many others, have answers as unique as the women who shared them here.

As a result, *Sex, Lies and Cosmetic Surgery* will be an insightful journey for the woman considering a change in appearance through cosmetic surgery.

David B. Sarwer, Ph.D.
Associate Professor of Psychology
Departments of Psychiatry and Surgery
The Edwin and Fannie Gray Hall Center for Human Appearance
University of Pennsylvania School of Medicine
Philadelphia, Pennsylvania
May 2006

Introduction

At one time I would have laughed with amusement at the mere suggestion that cosmetic surgery and sexuality were so inextricably intertwined, answered with a vehement "NO WAY", if asked my opinion. But now I know differently. In *Sex, Lies and Cosmetic Surgery* you will read many women's stories about sexuality as it relates to cosmetic surgery. These are the refreshingly honest stories women have shared with me during confidential interview sessions; stories from clients of well respected allied professionals (e.g. cosmetic surgery nurses, estheticians, psychologists, anesthesiologists) and yes, some personal stories of my own.

My suspicions began with my own experiences, but were confirmed the day I broached the topic of the relationship between sexuality and cosmetic surgery with Denise Thomas, the Manhattan Cosmetic Surgery Consultant whose pithy wisdom punctuates many chapters of this book. We experienced a binding of spirits during our second interview session, for she long knew what I only was beginning to discover - that cosmetic surgery is all about sexuality. Other women concurred. During interviews so personal that some asked to be identified only by fictitious first names, they told me so with words such as: "Now I'm the woman I always knew was hidden inside." Others shared feelings of renewal, with words such as: "I thought that time had passed me by, until I rediscovered my sexuality."

If you watched even a single episode of WABC TV's *Extreme Makeover*, you would have been struck by the heightened energy women exude after cosmetic surgery - the sensual quality that suddenly appears in their smiles, once awkward body movements now punctuated by feminine grace, averted eyes that suddenly sparkle with direct contact, flat personalities that begin to effervesce.

Through its primary theme of sexuality, this book raises our consciousness about many aspects of cosmetic surgery while destroying some long held myths and overly simplistic explanations. Is it really vanity that propels us or do we have deeper hidden motivations? Is it negative vibes which prompt us women to remain mute, to invent all manner of deception to shroud our surgical experiences behind a veil of secrecy, or is it embarrassment over our own ambivalent feelings?

Sex, Lies and Cosmetic Surgery is not a technical book about cosmetic surgery. A number of fine books, written by well-qualified physicians, are already on the market to meet those needs. But if you want to learn about the emotional underpinnings to cosmetic surgery, you need to listen to the voices of the many women who have contributed to this book - women who have already undergone some form of cosmetic surgery, nurses and estheticians who work along side them, and even some women who have avoided cosmetic surgery - for in this arena, they are the real experts. As *The Duchess of Dermis*, Michelle Martel, once commented: "Remember, plastic surgeons are tailors of the skin, not guardians of the soul." The many women who contributed to this book are the true guardians of our souls, for they have spoken so openly, revealing intimate details of their lives that they would never dare voice to their surgeons.

If you are perplexed by the soaring numbers of women who opt for cosmetic surgery, you need to read this book, for it will answer many of your questions and help clarify your perspective. If you are considering cosmetic surgery or have some ambivalent feelings, you should read this book, for it will give you an insider's view into things normally left unspoken. If you have already been there, have undergone some form of cosmetic surgery, you are likely to experience some jolts of recognition as you relate to many familiar moments. And if you are a repeat performer who has undergone multiple surgical procedures, *Sex, Lies and Cosmetic Surgery* has some non-judgmental thoughts for you to consider.

Finally, through its fresh insights, sound research and considerable empirical data, presented in a most readable, often entertaining format, this book is here for professionals who want a deeper understanding of the many emotional undercurrents experienced by cosmetic surgery patients,

The Epilogue that appears toward the end of this book tells my story, beginning with how I selected my surgeon, to those early days of post surgery healing and beyond. I did not start out as a savvy cosmetic surgery consumer, but I learned along the way that there is an intelligent approach to selecting a plastic surgeon. I hope my experiences will help women from as far away as Tallahassee to Chattanooga, Saskatchewan to Buenos Aires, choose wisely, because this critical decision can mean the difference between sublime surgical results and ruined appearances.

For the record, you should know that I had neither spoken to nor met Denise Thomas until long after my own cosmetic surgery. Although I value her knowledge, integrity and expertise and know that she gives her clients sound advice; this book is hardly a vehicle to promote her services. My only goal is to help you make sound decisions for yourself, so that if you decide to undergo cosmetic surgery, you can achieve the results you deserve.

Now I invite you to sit back, relax and enjoy the ride as you begin to read *Sex, Lies and Cosmetic Surgery.*

Lois W. Stern

✤ Please Note

Throughout this book I consistently refer to the plastic
surgeon as 'he' despite the fact that I am aware of many well
qualified, board certified female plastic surgeons. My sole
motivation is to avoid awkward s/he linguistics, not to
overlook the contributions of women to this field.

A Word About the End-of-Chapter Helpful Resources

At the conclusion of many chapters of this book,
you will see the words: *Helpful Resources*,
followed by either a CD: or a bell: 🔔
symbol.

The **Sex, Lies and Cosmetic Surgery** CD:
contains ten different self-evaluations forms, quizzes
and checklists, invaluable aids for the prospective
cosmetic surgery patient. The entire contents of this
CD are reproduced in print format at the back of this
book, beginning on Page 261; but you can order
them in their more convenient CD format at:

www.sexliesandcosmeticsurgery.com/

or by using the mail-in coupon at the end of this book

🔔 The numbered **Appendices** listed at the
conclusion of many chapters supplement the
contents of the specific chapter(s) in which they
appear. These appendices can be found in their own
section beginning on Page 300 at the back of this
book.

Chapter 1: Cosmetic Surgery – The Aphrodisiac Effect

The Short Story: The intimate relationship between physical appearance and sexuality

"Aphrodisiac: Arousing sexual desire"

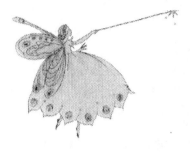

I love jokes that resonate with humor through an exaggeration of everyday possibility. Let me share a favorite – this one about one woman's out-of control behavior after her facelift:

> A woman decides to have a facelift for her birthday. She spends a lot of money, and is thrilled with the results. Several weeks later, she enters a cab and asks the driver: "How old do you think I am?"
>
> "About thirty-two", says the driver.
>
> "No, I'm actually forty-seven", the woman happily replies. Next she stops off at Starbucks for a quick latte. "How old do you think I am?", she asks the server.
>
> "Oh, I'd say about twenty-nine", he replies.

"No, I'm actually forty-seven", she says as she practically waltzes out the door. Now she is really feeling good about herself. While waiting in line to enter a museum, she poses her question once again, this time to the older gentleman standing behind her. "How old do you think I am?", she asks him.

"I've always had a fool proof way to determine a woman's age" says the gentleman, "but it requires me to put my hand inside your panties." Somewhat stunned, the woman stands in silence for a moment, but then recovers. She is feeling so jubilant that she says, "What the heck, go ahead." The man sticks his hand into her panties, lingers a bit until she says "Enough already", and then he quietly removes his hand.

"You're exactly forty-seven years old", he declares. "Why that's amazing", says the woman in some disbelief. "How did you determine that?" "Oh, that was easy" he replies with a satisfied grin. "I was standing behind you at Starbucks."

Most of us aren't so out of control after cosmetic surgery that we would allow a total stranger to insert his hand into our panties; but the point is, cosmetic surgery can be a pretty uplifting experience, with strong sexual overtones.

It didn't take long for Aphrodite, that Greek goddess of love and desire, to invade my life - an interesting side effect to my surgery. I questioned whether I was unique, or if cosmetic surgery impacted similarly upon the lives of other women. Did many experience a resurgence of sexuality? If so, did they dare reveal those feelings to themselves? Would they be willing to share such intimate details of their personal lives with a total stranger? I wondered how I could get those answers.

Then I happened upon an ad in New York magazine. Initially my eye was drawn to the photo of this woman who presented with unabashedly good looks. The words *Denise Thomas - Cosmetic Surgery Consultant* appeared beneath her photo; the words *Who's The Best Plastic Surgeon? How would you know?* were printed above.

Perhaps she could offer me some further insights to answer my many questions. I dialed her number to ask if she would be willing to talk with me.

Enter Denise Thomas

Denise's enthusiasm and obvious sense of fulfillment from her work enticed me further. She agreed to a series of interviews.

During our first session she told me some wonderful stories of ways her client's lives had changed after surgery. During our second session I returned to her earlier statement that after cosmetic surgery women come back and tell her how much more vital they feel, that women in their 50's and 60's tell her details of how their sex lives have improved.

I bit my tongue as I asked her if she could elaborate on this thought.

Denise said she was willing to do so as long as I understood that she would use fictitious names. She assured me that all her stories would be factual, but emphasized that she maintains confidential records and never reveals her clients' actual names. That established, Denise shared with candor.

She talked about several of her clients, but it wasn't until she spoke of **Cindy**, a fifty-two year old woman who said that before her cosmetic surgery she used to bury her face during sex because she felt so unattractive.

3

"Since my facelift, I'm no longer afraid to let my husband see that look of ecstasy that comes across my face while we're intimate.", she told Denise. "I feel so good about the way I look, that now I want to peer deep into his eyes instead of into his armpit."

At that moment I felt relief that this interview was taking place by phone rather than face-to-face. My jaw had gone slack, my mouth agape; but secretly I experience a sense of validation for some of my private feelings. "Women actually tell you these things?" I asked as I found my voice. "Of course. This is all about sexuality", she answered. "Denise, where were you when I needed you?" I laugh into the phone.

This is our bonding moment. It is also the moment when I realize I need to explore this unspoken relationship between cosmetic surgery and sexuality.

I was aware that sexuality was something people normally didn't speak about, especially in personal terms, and at first was reticent to pose such intimate probes, even on my anonymous questionnaire. But eventually my yearning to satisfy an innate curiosity triumphed over embarrassment and I began to interview other women.

As my interviews progressed, not only with Denise but with other women who had undergone cosmetic surgery, I was impressed by the honesty, sensitivity and total candor with which they spoke.

Other Women's Stories With Supporting Research

Katie, a forty-three year old hairstylist and Yoga teacher from Chicago, who had a breast lift and liposuction, hails from a large family of five adoring male siblings. During our interview, she confirmed this unspoken relationship between cosmetic surgery and sexuality.

"Several months after my surgery I posted a question on a women's Cosmetic Surgery Discussion Board: 'Why do I suddenly feel so sensual?' You should know that the average return rate for items listed on this discussion board is two and one half responses per posting, so you can imagine my surprise when I received thirty-seven responses within forty-eight hours. I printed them out. Here, I'll read you a few of them."

A woman named **Jolie** wrote: "Of course you do. You have just uncovered one of the unspoken benefits of cosmetic surgery." **Liza** expressed some sense of relief when she wrote: "Until I read your question, I could hardly admit that to myself, but now I see I'm not alone." But it was **Beth** who put it most succinctly with the words: "You're so right! Self-esteem is a great aphrodisiac."

Cosmetic Surgery often has a positive impact on sexual relationships. **Lauren,** an interior designer and active volunteer from Atlanta, Georgia, mirrors many of my own thoughts as she explains why she thinks that might be true.

> "It makes perfect sense that improving your personal appearance would have an impact on sexuality. The root of a woman's sensuality is in her brain. If she thinks she looks good and is appealing, desirable and attractive, naturally she will be more responsive sexually. She will also exude more confidence, which will only enhance her sexuality. All of her positive thoughts and feelings will also be further reinforced by her partner, friends and family, even perfect strangers."

After confirming anecdotal support for that link between physical appearance and sexuality, I began to look at the research. The first study I uncovered involved a population of one hundred ninety-two female college students. [1] These young women were asked to complete questions from the Snell Sexuality Scales (SS), a frequently used objective measurement of sexuality developed in the late 1980's, and subjectively rate themselves with an overall attractiveness score. They were unaware that simultaneously examiners were rating them discretely with an overall attractiveness score based on the same attractiveness scale.

This study concluded that a woman's subjective view of her face and body had the greatest impact on her sexual esteem, measured by dating history and sexual experience. In other words, her personal assessment of her attractiveness was the key factor to positive heterosexual relationships with more incidences of sexual activity.

Current research by both Cash et. al. and Weiderman clearly supports a positive link between body image (self-perceptions and self-attitudes toward one's overall facial and body appearance) and the quantity and quality of one's sexual activity. During such activity, they noted that persons with generally negative body image attitudes were:

> ". . . more likely to attend to those physical attributes they disliked, worry about their partner's perceptions, and try to cover or camouflage those body areas", (and concluded that) "these immediate body image experiences during sexual activity may adversely affect sexual desire, arousal, orgasm and satisfaction." **2   3**

I questioned whether that link transcended all age groups, as one might project that the significance of physical attractiveness declines with advancing age; but this next study suggests that, even in the elderly, body image is the key determinant in keeping sexuality alive. Surprisingly, Fooken concluded that health variables appeared of less significance than physical image in maintaining sexual interest and/or activity in a 60 + population. **4** After interviewing women whose ages range from the 20's through the 60's, I do believe that that link between physical appearance and sexuality transcends all age groups.

I recall the night I tuned in to the TV show, *Extreme Makeover*, to watch a crime scene investigative detective explain what happened to her as she aged. **Peggy** described how haggard she looked, how she wore the stress of her job on her face and felt it erode her spirit. We could see this for ourselves in the pre-surgery video footage, where at age forty-six, she already looked a good fifteen years older. When **Peggy** spoke about her failed marriage, she slipped in a very interesting comment. "It was me, not him. I had lost my sexuality." **5**

I couldn't help but notice the significance of her words, because when I watched **Peggy** after her makeover, it was quite evident she had rediscovered what she had previously lost.

During my interviews, I asked women of middle age and beyond if they experienced a sexual resurgence after surgery. I heard variations of this theme of renewal repeated in many of their stories. **Gail,** a professional singer, was one of them. This fifty-eight year old woman who, as a leisure time activity, likes nothing better than to curl up by a raging fire while enjoying the company of an intimate group of friends, spoke about her heightened sexuality after her facelift:

> "About six weeks after my surgery, my husband and I began to try out all the beds in our house – plus some other interesting places – mostly at my initiative. After awhile he had to remind me that I'm not twenty-one anymore even though I might like to be", she laughed. (And then she added this final thought that stirred my memory because I had done exactly the same thing.) "Another thought that strikes me - I threw out all my waist high, cotton underpants and bought all silky bikini pants in an array of gorgeous colors. Now that was a statement, wasn't it!"

More words of renewal came from **Anne**, a fifty-five year old registered nurse from Harrisburg, Pa.

> "I had a very Catholic upbringing so I'm not one to reveal juicy details about myself. But I will say, my facelift made me feel sexier, more flirtatious. For one thing, I initiate now. I never did much of that before. I nearly molested my husband."

Gina, a sixty-two year old retired elementary education teacher from San Diego, Ca., spoke about how she has become so much more focused on sex since her facelift. She told me that her husband recently commented: "You have become a much more sexual person since your cosmetic surgery. No matter what the topic, you seem to bring sex into the discussion. I never noticed you do that before."

Breasts give women much of their female identity so it is not surprising to hear stories about heightened sexuality after breast surgeries. This was the case for Denise's client, **Tanya**, a beautiful thirty-eight year old Russian woman whose breasts were deflated after two children. She confessed to Denise that she felt ashamed to get undressed in front of her husband, but after her breast lift, felt such a resurgence. "Now when my husband and I make love, I want the lights to remain on."

A twenty-nine year old respondent to my cosmetic surgery questionnaire, using the creative pen name, **Chesty**, wrote about her heightened sexuality following breast augmentation surgery:

> "It wasn't until after my surgery that I began to feel like a woman for the first time in my life. Before then I just felt too ashamed of my body to relax and enjoy sex. I didn't have my first orgasm until about six months after my surgery. Now it's a regular thing."

Research confirms what simple observations often tell us: all things being equal, men generally show a preference for fuller breasted women.

Singh and Young offer research to support the notion that when women's Waist-Hip Ratios are held constant, those with larger breasts were rated more attractive than women with a comparable WHR and smaller breasts. [6]

In another study, female patients reported that after breast augmentation surgery, their partners exhibited significantly greater interest in sexual activity and believed that their sexual relationship was significantly enhanced. [7] Although most studies conclude that women's primary motivation for cosmetic surgeries, including the two most frequently performed procedures, breast augmentation and lipoplasty, [8] is for improvement to self-esteem and body image and not to satisfy a romantic partner, the romantic partner's attitudes of an enhanced sexual relationship is likely to have a positive impact on the woman's sexuality as well.

We know that the perceptions others have of us impact our self-perceptions, so it is hardly a leap to surmise that a partner's attitude of an enhanced sexual relationship makes a woman feel more sexually desirable. You can feel the confluence of self-perception, partner's perception and heightened sexuality in this next story:

Nicole, a thirty-one year old woman from southern Florida who underwent breast augmentation after the birth of her second child, has appeared before the FDA as an advocate for a woman's right to choose breast augmentation. She leads support groups and is the creator and sole owner of the first and most active Internet resource for women undergoing breast augmentation procedures. She told me that after her surgery, she went out and bought sexy bras and the type clothes that she could only dream about wearing before.

"None of this was lost on my husband", said **Nicole**. "We had fun with it, like new toys. Even now, six years later, I still get such looks from him when I dress up – even if it's just a tight tank top. Our sex life is a million times better now because I feel so much more free. I'm so much less inhibited and initiate intimate situations more than I did in the past. When you feel sexier, more attractive, your partner picks up on that."

For **Tanya**, **Chesty** and **Nicole**, improving the overall appearance of their breasts clearly had a significant and positive impact on the quality of their lives, including intimacy.

If breasts are so important to a woman's identity, imagine how it feels to suddenly have one of them surgically removed. **Judy** gave me a poignant account of the loss of one of her breasts to breast cancer and her subsequent reconstructive surgery. Her story underscores just how deeply women define themselves by their anatomy.

"I always loved my body. I was really proud of it, and that made it easier for me to be comfortable with and take pleasure in the intimate aspects of my life. My breasts were particularly important to me and a very attractive part of my being.'

"The day I went to the hospital for a mastectomy, I felt like I was experiencing the death of part of my body. When I awakened from the anesthesia, the expander was already in place. I remember how self-conscious I was when I returned to work. I felt like people were staring at that one breast right through my clothing.'

"Six weeks later, after the implant was inserted, I remember looking in the mirror and finally feeling whole again. I took my surgeon's hands and said:

'Thank you for making me feel like a woman again.' The first thing I did was go to Victoria's Secret and buy the most sexy underpants, bras and nightgowns I could find. My nipple was reconstructed and two years later I had it tattooed. That was the final touch. Before the tattooing, when I looked in the mirror, my eye was always drawn to the reconstructed breast. Now, when I look in the mirror, I finally see balance and equality."

Our self-image is tied to many facets of our being: our families, our intellect, our achievements, our friendships, our worldly contributions. Although we might wish it were otherwise, physical attractiveness also impacts our self-image, which in turn impacts our sexuality.

In Wiederman & Hurst's study, we learn that thinner women who perceive their bodies as more attractive participate in more frequent and a greater variety of sex acts than those who are heavier and lacking that perception of attractiveness. For example, thinner women with positive self-perceptions of attractiveness were more likely to engage in any form of oral sex. [9]

I was not about to ask women specifics details concerning intimate aspects of their lives, but some shared spontaneously. In an article about self-image and sexuality, **Louise**, short for her home in Louisiana, explained further: "The less attractive I feel, the less I desire sex. If at all possible, I avoid sex (when feeling unattractive); however, if it should happen, I am unwilling to let go." [10]

A beautiful fifty-four year hairstylist named **Val** spoke about how even very temporary changes in self-perception influence her sexually:

"I personally don't feel attractive when I feel like I look old or fat. For me, the two things go together. If I don't feel attractive, I don't feel sensual and I'm just not interested in sex. But when I feel attractive, and most important, when my body is in good shape, well that's another story."

Physical Attractiveness: It's Link to Relationship Opportunities

There is a further side to physical attractiveness, self-image and sexuality. Not only does a woman who looks good often feel more confident and sexual, but studies continually equate looking good with a woman's *opportunities* for sexual liaisons. In studies conducted by Wiederman & Hurst, we learn that heavier and less facially attractive women were found to have fewer sexual experiences. **11** A study by Gortmaker, Sobol and Dietz, while reinforcing the above findings, further concluded that heavier, less facially attractive women hold similar attitudes toward sex and compare themselves as equally sexually capable as their slimmer, more facially attractive sisters. **12**

As much as our values may speak against this, cosmetic surgery does seem to improve dating and marital opportunities. Taking this thought one step further, in their journal article, *The Continuing Role of Physical Attractiveness in Marriage*, Margolin and White concluded that married men experience decreased sexual interest in wives who have gained weight or exhibited negative changes in body shape. **1**

> ". . . In the sexual domain, the importance of looks cannot be over estimated. People expect attractive people to be very popular, socially confidant and at ease. They also expect them to be sexually exciting, responsive, experienced and adventurous. Men expect beautiful women to have a high sex drive and prefer variety in sex." **14**

12

Dorothy Birnham, former Director of Voluntary Action on Long Island, a center sponsored by the American Red Cross, now lives in a popular retirement community in North Carolina. Although Dorothy never had cosmetic surgery, and explains the reasons for her choice in Chapter 8, *What Deters Us,* she willingly shared her observation about some of her friends enhanced marriage opportunities after their facelifts.

First she told a story about **Dani.**

> "After **Dani's** husband died, she knew she wanted to remarry and had her face done. She looked terrific afterwards. Now this is such a happy story. She went down to Texas to visit a friend. A male acquaintance of this friend saw Dani and subsequently asked for an introduction. Well, to make a long story short, now they are a happily married couple."

Although Dorothy concluded that she could not say that this facelift led **Dani** into the arms of a new husband, she thought it was possibly so. After all, it was her appearance that originally enticed this man to seek out an introduction. Dorothy spoke about four other friends who have had facelifts. In her words: "It worked out fine for each of them. They all look great." She told me that two of them were widowed at the time and have since remarried.

Then she thought about one further interesting story to share.

> "My friend **Sara** just had a lift for an unusual reason. Her husband is eighty-four years old and she still cares for him; but he is quite ill and she doesn't expect him to survive. She has prepared herself for the search for a new husband by planning ahead. She is sixteen years younger than her husband and wants to remarry."

Putting aside personal values, politics and philosophies - because Dorothy and I both acknowledged that we would like to see more value placed on other virtues - the fact remains that men are drawn to beauty. Cosmetic surgery enabled two of her widowed friends to enhance not simply their physical appearances but their marital opportunities as well. **Sara** just exemplified the epitome of planning ahead.

The subtle attitudes women receive from others – be they positive or negative – can become self-fulfilling prophesies. In the final analysis, that intimate relationship between physical appearance and sexuality seems born of self-image, opportunity and attitudes projected by sexual partners.

Helpful Resources

See also the following end-of-book helpful resources pertinent to information found in this chapter.

CD Part A: Test Your Sexuality Quotient (SQ).

☼ **Appendix 1: Meet Denise Thomas**

☼ **Appendix 2: The Anatomy of an Interview** (Structuring my personal interviews)

☼ **Appendix 3: My Cosmetic Surgery Questionnaire**

☼ **Appendix 8: Personal Profiles** (More about the people whose names appear in this chapter)

☼ **Appendix 9: Additional Stories for Chapter 1**

Footnotes

1. Wiederman M. and Hurst, S., "Body size, physical attractiveness and body image among young adult women." <u>Journal of Sex Research</u>. Vol. 35 Issue 3. (August 98): 272.

2. Cash TF. Maikkula CL. and Yammiya Y. "Baring the body in the bedroom: body image, sexual self-schemas, and sexual functioning among college women and men." <u>Elect J Human Sex</u> [serial online]. Vol.7. Available at http://www.ejhs.org/volume7/bodyimage.html accessed (June 29, 2004).

3. Weiderman MW. "Body image and sexual functioning." In: Cash TF. Pruzinsky T. eds. <u>Body Image: A Handbook of Theory, Research, and Clinical Practice</u>. New York: Guilford Press. (2002): 287-294.

4. Fooken I. "Sexuality in the later years-the impact of health and body image in a sample of older women." <u>Patient Education and Counseling</u>. 23(3). (1994): 227-233.

5. WABC TV: Extreme Makeover. Sept. 25, 2003.

6. Singh D. and Young RK. "Body weight, waist-to-hip ratio, breasts and hips: role is judgments of female attractiveness and desirability for relationships". <u>Ethol Sociobiol</u>. (1995). 16: 483-507.

7. Kilman P. Sattler J. and Taylor J. "The impact of augmentation mammaplasty: A follow-up study. " Department of Psychology at the University of South Carolina. (1986).

8. Statistic compiled by the American Society for Aesthetic Plastic Surgery (2005).

9. Wiederman M. and Hurst S. "Body size, physical attractiveness and body image among young adult women." <u>Journal of Sex Research</u>. Vol. 35 Issue 3 (August 98): 272.

10. Hamburger A. and Hall H. "Beauty Quest". <u>Psychology Today</u>.

22.5 (May 1988): 28(5).

11. Wiederman M. and Hurst S., "Body size, physical attractiveness and body image among young adult women." Journal of Sex Research. 35.3 (August 98): 272.

12. Gortmaker S. Must A. Pen-in J. Sobol A. and Dietz W. "Social and economic consequences of overweight in adolescence and young adulthood. " New England Journal of Medicine. 329: (1987): 1008-1012.

13. Margolin L and White L. "The continuing role of physical attractiveness in marriage." Journal of Marriage and the Family. 49. (1987): 21-27.

14. Etcoff N. Survival of the Prettiest – The Science of Beauty. Doubleday. (1999): 50.

The Short Story

"Your facelift was a good investment for both of us", says that guy I've been living with for over 35 years.

"Metamorphosis: A striking alteration in appearance, character or circumstance"

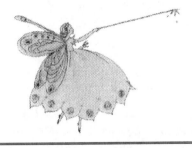

How do I know so much about cosmetic surgery and sexuality? Here is my up front and personal story.

About one year prior to surgery, I was seated opposite my new internist, answering questions about my medical history. This was our first meeting so I surely was unprepared for this personal probe: "Are you sexually active?" he asked. My eyes immediately became riveted to the floor, as I looked for an opening to swallow me whole. None materialized. I lifted my head slightly to meet his gaze and noted that he was waiting patiently for an answer. "Well, that depends on your definition of active", I finally mustered.

He wasn't about to let me off the hook so readily. "You have a partner? A husband?" he said, in a half statement, half

19

questioning tone. "Yes, but we've been married for over thirty-five years", I say. "It isn't exactly like we're newlyweds anymore." He let that thought drop, but I didn't. I left his office feeling unsettled.

"You jerk", I said to myself. "Why do you feel a need for full disclosure? Couldn't you have just said 'yes' and left it at that?" But I must admit, I felt a bit wistful, reflective. Then I tucked those thoughts safely away.

If I were asked that question today, I would answer very differently.

It began at the end of my first week post surgery. I got out of the shower, wrapped in an oversize towel and danced around Ken in our bedroom singing: "I feel pretty." It was such a good feeling - so hard to explain. I just felt so good.

Several days later, I was talking to **Linda Gottlieb**, Dr. K. . .'s nurse practitioner, about some of these feelings when Dr. K. . . knocked on the door and entered. "I want to hug you", I said. And I did. He hugged me back without embarrassment. I thought about this interchange later. I felt that old me reemerging – the one with an element of spontaneity that had become subdued over the years. "Is there such a strong link between physical presence and outward response?" I wondered.

I discovered **Michelle Martel,** a talented esthetician - so enthusiastic and knowledgeable about her field, that her passion became contagious. Before long I was thoroughly immersed in this altogether new project called skin care. She taught me so much about skin, a topic that up until now hadn't piqued my slightest interest. Now it was more like a daily ritual.

As my complexion began to take on a more translucent glow it, only added to the inner glow I was feeling. My happiness barometer was inching skyward.

I initiated several more self-improvement projects soon after cosmetic surgery. I had a head start on weight loss during those early post surgery days when it had been so hard to chew and swallow. I grew accustomed to smaller portions then and maintained that pattern. Not a diet per se – just increased amounts of fruits, veggies and water. Smaller portions of everything else.

I added forty minutes of early morning treadmill exercises to my daily routine. That combination of exercise and healthy eating helped melt away those few extra pounds. I could feel my clothes loosening around my waist and hips. I liked the feel of repossessing my slimmer body.

I wondered if my new chin would afford me more hairstyle options. I was ready for a softer, more feminine style. I let my hair grow out of its severely cropped, layered cut. I no longer fought my natural curl, but instead learned to scrunch with gel, dry with a diffuser, to achieve a more appealing effect. Subtle changes perhaps, but ones that delivered a feeling of femininity I was beginning to savor. I was so high on life, actually elated. I didn't want to lose that feeling, although I still hadn't a clue from whence it came. I was heading straight for the stratosphere.

I see **Michelle** six weeks post surgery and share some of my conflicted feelings.

> "I'm a little taken aback by my vanity," I say to her. "I never thought my appearance was so important to me. On the one hand I am so happy with the results, but I feel ashamed that these surface things should make me feel so happy."

She asks me why this troubles me.

> "Well, I've always hated the word vanity, I begin. "It

just goes against my value system. Right away I think of people who are shallow, lacking in substance, superficial, and I know I'm not any of those things. None of those words fit the self-image I have worn for a lifetime. So I don't understand why all these exterior changes are making me feel so good."

"It's not vanity", she explains. "It's more a girl thing. Most guys just wouldn't understand. You spent a lot of years devoted to your career. Now it's time for you. You're still all the other things you always were."

I wondered what the difference was between "a girl thing" and vanity. I still didn't get it, but why question such elation? I was smiling day and night, whacking that tennis ball across the court, humming to my computer, dancing around the house with flailing arms and wriggling hips, singing Mamma Mia above the highest volume on my CD player. My happiness gauge had reached max. I knew I was electrically charged, way up there in the ionosphere, but who needs to analyze such 'feel good' feelings?

Then one day the core to my metamorphic feelings begins to creep into consciousness. It's about three weeks after my 'girl thing' conversation with Michelle. Ken and I are seated in his office library, working on papers regarding my mom's nursing home placement. He picks up the phone to respond to a client's inquiries. I listen to his responses - so intelligent, balanced and filled with genuine caring.

We continue with our paper work. Another client enters unannounced. They move to the back office, but I hear his tone. I think to myself, *this man is so lacking in greed, so motivated to do right by his clients, not himself.* When we finish our paper work and we are alone again, I say, "You know, if I never knew you, if you weren't my husband, I would just hope and pray that I could find an attorney who

would take such genuinely good care of me."
But the rest of the day I am thinking much more. . . .

My thoughts take me back to Columbia College, to the days when we first met. I was nineteen. He was twenty. He was the business manager of the school paper, the Columbia Spectator. I used to admire how he tackled deadlines and challenges, the dedication he showed, the humor he brought to so many situations.

I remembered how I slackened off during the first semester of Economics and then panicked the day before the midterm. He stayed up with me the entire night to help me cram. How much I appreciated all his kindness and support.

I felt a warm glow as I recalled the evenings we splurged on a horse drawn carriage ride through Central Park, just to satisfy our youthful yearnings. Why was I suddenly flooded with all these thoughts? It began to strike me that the things that made me fall in love with this man so many years ago, were the very things that made me feel so special about him at this moment.

Nothing had changed. Yet everything seemed changed. I was shaken from my complacency. Finally I was able to put a label to my mounting emotionality, my continually soaring happiness barometer. *So this is what it's all about*, I thought with amazement. *Sexuality is the key.*

I couldn't wait for Ken to get home that night.

Well, I know what you want to ask. The short answer is "yes". The question of "why" is harder to pinpoint. Why this resurgence of admiration, appreciation, even passion at this stage of our lives? Suddenly I feel the power of self-esteem, its connectiveness to sexuality. I realize that all my little self-improvement projects were moving me in that direction. I guess I had arrived.

Four months have passed. It's early summer now. After a weekend with a particularly full social calendar, we are driving home from an outdoor concert. Ken shares some of his thoughts from these last forty-eight hours: how happy he felt just watching me walk toward him from across the lawn, how pretty I looked on the dance floor, how confidant I appear. He explains that it isn't so much how I *look* as it is my renewed exuberance that he finds so attractive.

My smile says it all as I snuggle closer to him. I confess how truly wonderful I feel, how happy I am with our lives together.

I'm lying in bed that next morning in a kind of revelry, when I feel Ken stir beside me. I roll toward him and see that his eyes are starting to open. "You know, I was just thinking", I say dreamily. "When people make love, it's pretty much a reflection of who they are . . . . You're so caring, unselfish."

He takes this all in without comment. I prop myself up on one elbow to get some eye contact here. "Ken", I ask. "How would you rate me as a sex partner?" In all our years together, I had never asked him that question. But at this very moment I really wanted to know. I was feeling like a ten. Maybe I just wanted to hear him say: "Lo, you're a ten."

But he doesn't answer with a number. Instead he puts his arms around me and buries his nose in my hair. "You're fine. You're absolutely fine", he says in muffled tones. "What are you so worried about? . . .
Lo, do you really think it's necessary to talk about all this?"

An hour later, he kisses me good-bye before he leaves for his office. I tell him that I have a follow-up appointment with Dr. K . . . that morning. "Well, do say thank you to Dr. K . . .", he says with a wink. "Tell him I think your facelift was a very good investment for both of us."

Chapter 3: What Can You Expect After Cosmetic Surgery

The Short Story: The Synergistic Effect

"Synergy: A total effect that is more than the sum of its parts"

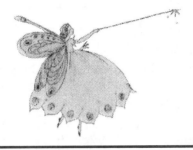

Animal behaviorist often refer to their subjects' sexuality as animal *courtship,* including in this term all behaviors that precede and accompany the sex act for the purpose of conception of young. **1** It is interesting to note current research suggesting that historically, the physical features impacted by testosterone production in adult males and high estrogen levels in women were deemed sexually attractive in part due to the reproductive potential these very characteristics signaled. **2**

But today humans do not use their sexuality exclusively, nor for that matter, primarily, for procreation. Much of our display of sexuality is tied up in presentation: the way we walk, carry ourselves, wear our hair, dress, smile, in our mannerisms, gestures and words. All of these displays are used to attract others to us and can culminate in sexual acts, but often the ultimate goal is simply to attract and feel attractive.

So when we speak about women being more sexual after cosmetic surgery, we shouldn't conclude that post surgery all women suddenly transform themselves into sexual Olympiads. What it does mean, however, is that after cosmetic surgery women might project a more sensual image, because that is one way cosmetic surgery is likely to transform their feelings about themselves.

I can explain this feeling best by sharing a personal story about one of my social interactions in the early months after my cosmetic surgery:

I've always had a bit of quirkiness to my personality, but normally keep it in check, save responses with sexual innuendo for Ken and my closest women friends. But I noticed that after my cosmetic surgery, that seemed to change a bit. Here is one example.

I was eating dinner with a group of friends one evening. Burt, a generally expansive man both in personality and body language, was seated diagonally across from me. Before coffee, he stretched his legs out under the table until one of his shoes was resting against my inner thigh.

I know he was totally unconscious of its new found resting place and I easily could have disengaged by shifting my position slightly. But instead, I looked him in the eye and said, "Burt, would you mind removing your foot from between my legs."

Undaunted, he came back at me with, "Oh, my, if only I were wearing my sandals tonight." I kind of surprised myself, but at the same time amused both me and my friends by continuing the repartee: "Do you think I would have asked you to move your foot so quickly if you were wearing sandals?" I answered coyly.

We all laughed, especially his wife Vivian, who took this verbal interchange exactly as intended. How wonderful to feel comfortable enough to express such feelings with really good friends.

The point to my story is this:
When I asked other women if they felt altered beyond surface cosmetic changes after their surgeries, I offered them some examples as:

a) Younger, more energetic
b) More outgoing, friendlier
c) Happier, more content
d) Prettier
e) More self-confident
f) More sensual
g) More flirtatious
h) Same as before
(i) – (m) Opposite statements from the first seven:
Less friendly, Less happy or less content, Less sensual, Less flirtatious, etc.

If I had responded to my own question about altered feelings that evening, I would have selected statements (a) – (g).

These feelings don't necessarily translate into being more sexually active, but as we have seen, after cosmetic surgery this is sometimes a reality.

Looking again at the animal kingdom, we see that the male is often the courtship aggressor. The male peacock and sage grouse posture in front of the female to show off their spectacular plumage. Many of the male garden birds use their songs to attract females of their species.

Similarly, in many human cultures, the male normally has been the sexual aggressor. But in western societies this is not always the norm. Attraction might be a mutual endeavor or the female might be the one to initiate male attention and interest.

Within some sectors of the animal kingdom we can find counter points to the male-as-aggressor. The iguana is one such example.

> "The female iguana leads the male on a merry chase. While making small physical signs of her readiness to mate, she dashes off tail high and taunts him until his passion can no longer be contained." **3**

The female vulture demonstrates her sexual aggression more subtly, but it is still observable.

> "Through acts of coyness, she stimulates and encourages the potential male mate." **4**

After cosmetic surgery, some women seem to reflect the behavior of the female vulture or iguana, becoming more sexually assertive, initiating and stimulating their partners moreso than prior to their surgeries.

One additional similarity between animal and human sexuality can be found in the special devices and structures that aid their courtship. Some animals have vividly colored bare patches, combs, body parts that can be pumped up with air or blood to stimulate the mate. **5**

> "The concept of and appreciation of beauty is a function of sexual stimulation in animals " **6**

It is no less so in humans where the concept of and appreciation of beauty serve as sexual stimulants. Many women find that after their surgeries they have a heightened interest in adornments. They might dress differently, change the color or style of their hair, use more skin care or cosmetic products.

Whether women express their sexuality with the subtlety of a vulture or in the spirited manner of an iguana, whether it is a conscious behavior or an unconscious display, it is a deeply ingrained part of our being. As **Judy**, the woman who underwent reconstructive breast surgery commented, "I think sex is a thread that runs deeper within us than any of us realize."

Further Impacts to Cosmetic Surgery

As my interviews progressed, I discovered that many women experienced altered feelings about themselves after cosmetic surgery, and expressed that thought in various ways.

Nicole, the young mother you met in Chapter 1, *Cosmetic Surgery –The Aphrodisiac Effect,* who created a breast augmentation Internet support site after her own surgery, explained that although she had always been in shape and took care of her appearance, she somehow never felt complete. But after surgery, she described feeling reborn. "It affected my whole life. I'm happier, more self-confident and that has had a trickle down effect on many other facets of my life."

Nicole realizes that the reasons breast augmentation made such a change for her are more complex than just appearance, but that it somehow completed her by giving her something that she felt had been missing. "Even six years later I still look at my breasts when I shower or get undressed and think: *Wow, they are pretty.*"

> ". . . Body image, which is intimately linked to appearance, is an integral component of one's psyche and remains a powerful motive throughout our lives."
> 7

Body image can make a huge difference in the way we feel about ourselves and that image can impact in many ways, including our sexuality. This was especially true for **Chesty**, the twenty-nine year old woman you met in Chapter 1, *Cosmetic Surgery – The Aphrodisiac Effect,* who was unable to respond sexually until after her breast augmentation surgery. She expressed this same feeling of alteration when she wrote: "It's like someone took a magic wand and changed my personal nightmare into a dream come true."

Perhaps those of us who always felt some body part was insufficient – be it a chin or breasts - are more deeply impacted by our surgeries.

Outcomes of several contemporary studies support the validity of the strong link between physical appearance and self-esteem. For example, in a 1997 Body Image Survey, four thousand people were asked: "How many years of your life would you trade to achieve your weight goals?" **8** Astoundingly, twenty-four percent of the women respondents said they would give up more than three years of their life to achieve their ideal weight. Fifteen percent said they would sacrifice more than five years. This extreme proposed trade off underscores the significance of physical appearance to many women.

If you think back to Chapter 1, *Cosmetic Surgery – The Aphrodisiac Effect,* where **Nicole**, **Peggy**, **Tanya** and others talked about enriched sexual relationships after cosmetic surgery, you know that was a reality for them, as it was for **Kelly,** a fifty-two year old woman too shy to reveal details that might identify her, but spoke about her relationship with her husband after her breast augmentation and eyelift.

> "We are just living a more exciting life now, flying to Europe, going to nice restaurants and theatre, and having fun. My husband is probably more thrilled than I am. He feels that I am in such nice shape that he wants to show me off. I've become more sexually assertive and he really likes that. He encourages me to wear tight dresses and even wants me to have more

surgery, but right now I'm happy with how I look – don't want to go overboard."

Nancy, a forty-three year old who had a breast reduction, reported a similar relationship boost after her surgery.

> "My husband was extremely supportive. When I told him I wanted to have cosmetic surgery and explained my reasons, he encouraged me. He took money out of his retirement fund because he said he wanted me to feel special. Both of us had upbeat attitudes before, but now we feel like we're on a second honeymoon."

Enhanced relationships are a wonderful fringe benefit to cosmetic surgery for some. But as you will learn in Chapter 9, *Secrecy, Deception and Lies,* there are situations where the outcome is quite the reverse.

What else can you expect after cosmetic surgery? From my interviews with other women, I found that increased confidence and a more positive attitude were high on the list.

"I feel more at ease, more confident talking to people. I just feel good", said the fifty-seven year old tall, slender woman seated opposite me at a Long Island diner. Introduced through a friend, **Diane** and I shared soup and salad as we talked. Her outgoing personality engaged me instantly. I needed no further elaboration to the few words she used to describe herself: "I am generous in my friendships."

She told me that since her facelift, when she gets dressed and looks in the mirror, she feels happy. "It gives me a more positive attitude. I notice subtle differences in the way I project my personality. Now I can look someone right in the eye. When you feel confident and good about yourself, other people relate that way to you."

Fran Orgovan, a skilled clinical esthetician who instructs other estheticians in advanced skin care techniques, made similar observations. In her years of experience working with her clients both before and after their surgeries, **Fran** has observed that women who already are confident, get more confidence afterwards. "They don't just smile after surgery - they beam, and dress differently too, like they want to flaunt their newly discovered sexuality."

Fran believes cosmetic surgery is an event that just enhances women who have an underlying sense of self to begin with, by making them feel more beautiful and happier than they were before.

That extra burst of self-confidence fostered life enhancements for **Rose**, a thirty-seven year old clinical psychotherapist who began to enter body building competitions after her rhinoplasty surgery.

> "At each competition I was on display before a large audience and would be photographed. I never would have been able to do that with my old nose. I would have been much too self-conscious."

The glow on her face reflected **Fran's** description of some of her clients, for **Rose** is another woman who doesn't just smile – she beams.

Greater visibility is one more realistic expectation after cosmetic surgery. A disturbing reality for many women as they age is that society increasingly treats them as nonentities. **Gail**, the professional singer who prefers quiet evenings by a fire and intimate social gatherings, spoke about daily episodes of warmth she now receives from total strangers.

> "That veil of invisibility definitely has melted away. I see looks of receptiveness, hear comments about my high energy and enthusiasm, am told that I radiate an aura of joy. Men are right out there in their expressions of approval, both strangers and friends

alike. And I am here to tell you that that affirmation feels good! This from a woman who has never looked for extra curricular activity, is such a monogamous person at heart, that it still means the most to me when it comes from John."

Women without partners sometimes undergo cosmetic surgery with expectations of attracting someone new. You can see from Chapter 1, *Cosmetic Surgery, The Aphrodisiac Effect,* where **Dorothy Birnham** shared stories of three of her widowed friends, and in the next chapter where **Denise Thomas** shares stories about some of her clients, that at times cosmetic surgery does helps women succeed in meeting new partners.

When you read Chapter 4, *Preferential Treatment for the Pretty Ones,* you will discover that marital opportunities are significantly enhanced for physically attractive women. But I suspect there is also some synergy involved here, because when you feel more confident, reach out to others with more direct eye contact, radiate an inner glow and an outward smile, you have created a package of ingredients that make you a more magnetic woman, tend to attract others to you.

If you have cosmetic surgery, will your newly refreshed appearance send men racing to your doorstep? Probably not. But that new physical you coupled with your newly invigorated attitude create an image more difficult to ignore.

If you are looking to add a meaningful relationship to your life, as a first step you need to get noticed before some lucky person strives to get to know you more intimately. Ultimately it will be your personality, interests, talents, accomplishments, values . . . the stuff that's inside, that cement a lasting relationship. Beauty only opens the door. The rest is up to you.

In an ideal world, surface appearances probably wouldn't count, but in the world in which we live, the reality is that one's appearance does make a difference.

What can you expect after cosmetic surgery? Like **Kelly** and **Diane**, you may very well wake up in the morning with a higher energy level, with more enthusiasm as you go through the day. You might feel a bit more bouncy, show more lighthearted humor in your everyday interactions, become more deeply involved in whatever you love to do.

Does this renewed zest for life turn you into a more sexual person? Possibly yes. It did for **Nicole** and **Chesty**, but this should be no surprise to anyone. Young women, suddenly gifted with beautiful new breasts, would likely become more sexual. But as you saw in Chapter 1, *Cosmetic Surgery, The Aphrodisiac Effect*, even more mature women who have had only facial surgery, often become more sexual after cosmetic surgery. Think of **Gail**, the fifty-eight year old woman whose husband had to remind her that she wasn't twenty-one anymore. Think of **Gina**, the sixty-two year old woman whose husband observed that after her facelift she seemed so much more focused on sexual content. Think of me.

But cosmetic surgery is not a pure aphrodisiac. If you have sexual problems, have never been an enthusiastic participant, don't count on cosmetic surgery to reverse the pattern. We will return to this topic in later chapters.

What else can you expect after cosmetic surgery? I suspect that there are some health related benefits to looking good. I know I have become more focused on diet and exercise and five years later, still have maintained my routine.

I identified with **Diane** completely when she told me that she never did so much for herself before. "My husband used to encourage me to get some form of exercise. 'At least take walks', he used to say. I found a million excuses not to do it. Now I'm so focused on keeping my body healthy. I go to the gym, use a personal trainer, watch my weight and the inches."

Anne, the registered nurse from Harrisburg, Pa., told a very similar story. "I started an exercise program to keep in shape. Now I walk or run on a regular basis. I even bought a health club membership as a Christmas present for my husband and me." **Carol**, a retired math teacher whom you will officially meet in Chapter 7, *What Propels Us?* concurred: "My surgery was an incentive to keep working out, for the body has to keep up with the face."

Fran Orgovan made one further interesting observation:

> "When women come to me after cosmetic surgery, they never seem to complain about menopause symptoms, pains in their legs or backs. Somehow once their attitudes change, they feel younger and they act younger."

I do believe positive self-esteem can impact on our physical well-being in much the same manner as the exercise routines we initiate. This mind/body connection has been well validated in the past. Positive self-esteem may keep us healthier in and of itself. It also frequently motivates us to take proactive steps for ourselves. During my interviews, I was struck by the number of women who mentioned their involvement in either home or gym based exercise programs following cosmetic surgery. This is almost predictable, since once a woman is looking good and feeling good about her appearance; she tends to initiate steps to maintain or improve her health.

Because I was aware of this renewed focus on good health after cosmetic surgery, I wasn't surprised to read the results of the Mayo Clinic study that follows: **9**

In this study the Mayo Clinic tracked two hundred and fifty female patients who had facelifts at an average age of 60.4 years. At the time of follow-up over twenty years later, sixty-six percent of these women were still alive, at an average age of eighty-four years. By statistical comparison, the facelift patients had a life expectancy more than ten years greater than that of the general female population.

This study does not claim to prove a cause-effect relationship between facelifts and longevity. But it does support findings from two other studies that suggest that cosmetic surgery patients are strongly dedicated to health and fitness. **10 11**

As Mark Jewell, MD, President of the Board of Directors of the prestigious ASAPS (American Society for Aesthetic Plastic Surgery) for its 2005-2006 term explains:

> ". . . patients who have a facelift generally have a greater-than-average commitment to maintaining their overall health and fitness. This can easily translate into living longer."

What I have learned from my experiences with cosmetic surgery is that its impacts are going to vary, as each person's individuality is bound to come into play. But clearly its benefits can extend far beyond what appears on the rejuvenated face or newly sculpted body. With synergistic effect, the total outcome can be greater than the sum of its parts, enriching one's life and feelings of well-being. The benefits may sit at the very core of how you feel about yourself. Because when you are healthier, feeling good about yourself and projecting a positive image, you are likely to be more fully optimized in many facets of your life.

But occasionally a cosmetic surgery patient experiences surgical results that do not mesh well with her expectations. This woman would likely select from amongst statements i-m (less happy, less outgoing, less sensual) on the Cosmetic Surgery Questionnaire noted earlier in this chapter. As most every plastic surgeon already knows, it takes more than quality surgery for a successful outcome. Sound motivations, realistic expectations and a healthy mental outlook are the other keys to patient satisfaction.

Helpful Resources

See also the following end-of-book helpful resources pertinent to information found in this chapter.

 CD Part B: Test Your Self-Esteem

Appendix 8: Personal Profiles
(More about the people whose
names appear in this chapter)

Appendix 9: Additional Stories for Chapter 3

Footnotes

1. McFarland D. ed. <u>The Oxford Companion to Animal Behavior</u>. Oxford University Press. (1982): 106.

2. Mueller U. and Mazur A. "Facial dominance in *Homo Sapiens* as honest signaling of male quality". <u>Behavioral Ecology</u>. (1997) 8: 569-579.

3. Caras R. ed. <u>Animal Courtships</u>. Westover Publishing Company. (1972): 50.

4. Caras R. ed. <u>Animal Courtships</u>. Westover Publishing Company. (1972): 50.

5. Cloudsley-Thomas J.L. <u>Animal Behavior</u>. Macmillan. NY (1960): 107.

6. Cloudsley-Thomas J.L. <u>Animal Behavior</u>. Macmillan. NY (1960): 108.

7. Cash TF. "Body image and plastic surgery." In. <u>Psychological Aspects of Reconstructive and Cosmetic Plastic Surgery: Clinical, Empirical and Ethical Perspectives</u>. Lippincott, Williams and Wilkens. (Sept. 2005): 37-59.

8. Garner DM. "The body image survey." <u>Psychology Today</u>. 30. 1. (Feb. 97): 30(18).

9. Smith L. and Finical S. "Facelift: does looking younger help you live longer?" Mayo Clinic Study. (July 9, 2001).

10. Didie ER. and Sarwer DB. <u>J Women's Health</u>. (2003): 241-253.

11. Sarwer DB. Wadden TA Pertschuk MJ and Whitaker LA. "Body image dissatisfactionand body dysmorphic disorder in 100 cosmetic surgery patients". Plastic and Reconstructive Surgery. 101(1998):1644-1649.

Chapter 4: Preferential Treatment
For the Pretty Ones

The Short Story:

When physically attractive people receive more than their share

"Preferential: The act or principle of giving advantage to some over others"

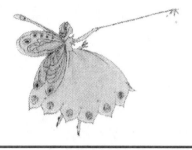

In his analysis of a 'body-in-society' view, Cash explains:

> "Whether due to bio-evolutionary 'pre-wiring',
> cultural socialization, or people's interactions with
> each other, there is little doubt that physical
> appearance can exert both subtle and profound effects
> on human relations, from infancy to old age, and
> from the bedroom to the boardroom." **1**

People are attracted to beauty. We are often quick to surmise that this attraction is born of social conditioning, but the outcomes from several studies contradict this thought.

Psychologists Langlois et al. collected hundreds of slides of people's faces and had adults rate them for attractiveness.

When she presented her slides to three and six month old babies, the infants stared significantly longer at the faces which adults had previously rated as particularly attractive. Neither sex, race nor age was a determining factor. **2**

At the British Association Festival of Science held in late Sept. 2004, Dr. Alan Slater, a developmental psychologist at the University of Exeter, presented work showing that babies as young as five hours old invariably spent more time looking at photographs of attractive faces rather than those rated by adults as not so attractive. **3**

These two studies speak against the belief that we are culturally conditioned to recognize human beauty. Even tiny babies seem innately drawn to it.

This attraction to beauty continues as babies grow and mature. In a study of four year old children who were rated for physical attractiveness by a group of adults and rated for popularity by professionals who regularly worked with these children, it turned out that in most cases the best looking children were also the most popular. **4**

I asked **Denise** to comment on the subject of preferential treatment for physically attractive people. She shared feedback she gets from her clients, beginning with observations about their increased visibility after cosmetic surgery. Women tell her that suddenly the doorman runs to help them with their packages or that they are being given better seats at restaurants and then served more attentively.

Zena, a forty-eight year old former fashion model, told me a story about the favored service she received from a Las Vegas attendant several months after her facelift.

> "When my husband and I walked into the theatre, we noticed that ushers were seating people toward the rear of the auditorium and then accepting tips for better placements. When it was our turn, the usher

looked me right in the eye, smiled and said: 'Follow
me. I have special seats for my beautiful women.'
Then he led us down the aisle to two orchestra seats
about five rows from the stage."

Dr. David Sarwer, Associate Professor of Psychology at the
University of Pennsylvania School of Medicine, explains it
this way:

"Research has repeatedly demonstrated the
importance of physical appearance in daily life.
Persons who are considered physically attractive
receive preferential social treatment in virtually every
situation examined to date including education,
employment, medical care, legal proceedings, and
romantic encounters. Clearly, in our society
appearance matters." **5**

Denise spoke about financial benefits that come to some of
her clients after their surgeries. "They tell me they are
offered better work positions and given promotions more
readily."

She shared the story of a client photographer she called
Pamela, who at age fifty-three, when she first came to Denise
for cosmetic surgery advise, was thirty pounds overweight,
with bushy hair and hooded eyes. "Although she was a very
talented photographer, she just couldn't get past that first
interview. Her career was stagnant." After cosmetic surgery,
Pamela lost thirty pound and restyled her hair. "Not only
does she look beautiful", said Denise, "but her career has
blossomed. She is now a very successful photographer. You
see, we are all attracted to beauty."

Denise explained that it all starts with self-esteem, because
when you look better and are more out there, feeling so good
about yourself, it's bound to show and be noticed by others.
She believes these feelings have a trickle down effect that
permeates other facets of people's lives.

A Ph.D. psychologist who designed and implemented a Body Image Survey for Psychology Today, reiterates Denise's thoughts:

> "Our body perceptions, feelings and beliefs govern our life's plan – whom we meet, whom we marry, the nature of our interactions, our day to day comfort level. Indeed our body is our personal billboard, providing others with first-- and sometimes only-- impressions." **6**

Rose, the clinical psychologist you first met in Chapter 3, *What Can You Expect After Cosmetic Surgery?*, experienced a career boost after her rhinoplasty (nose job).

> "When new clients call my office, they ask my office manager what I look like. Am I old or young? And since I had my nose fixed, I feel more confidant knowing that I look attractive."

Rose commented that perhaps if a therapist is knock down gorgeous, it might be intimidating; but that otherwise, a nice appearance is definitely an asset.

She is aware that her improved appearance has helped her become a more effective therapist, a part of the trickle down effect Denise mentioned earlier.

Katie, the forty-three year old hairstylist whom you met in Chapter 1, *Cosmetic Surgery, The Aphrodisiac Effect,* who posted a question on a women's Cosmetic Surgery Discussion Board about why she was feeling so sensual since her surgery, shared subtle differences she has noted in the way her friends' husbands treat her now.

> "I'm thinking of one man who for years would greet me with a peck on the cheek. Now he goes for my lips each time we meet. I think it's an unconscious

thing, but it certainly tells me that he finds me more alluring."

You met **Gina** earlier in Chapter 1, *Cosmetic Surgery, The Aphrodisiac Effect* and Chapter 3, *What Can You Expect After Cosmetic Surgery?,* the woman whose husband noticed that since her facelift, she 'jumps to attention' whenever anything sex related comes on the TV screen. **Gina** recalled this episode where she received more attention from a male friend than customary.

> "One of my friend's husbands bumped into me at the supermarket several months after my facelift. His first reaction was, 'I love your new hair style.' I thanked him and explained that I needed a haircut badly, actually had an appointment for later that afternoon. 'No, don't cut it – I love this hair style on you', he practically shouted as he continued to look at me admiringly."

> "Then he shook his head and added, 'I don't know, Gina, you keep getting younger while the rest of us keep on aging.' My experience has been that men notice and comment, whereas women notice but are more likely to remain silent."

Lucy, a fifty-four year old whom you'll meet again in Chapter 7, *What Propels Us,* commented that since her facelift, she notices that she is singled out for more hugs and good-natured bantering from men. As an example, she told this story of what happened during intermission at a concert she recently attended.

> "Several of us headed toward the bar. One of my friend's husbands put his arm around my waist and said to the bartender: 'See this young woman. She's an Iranian Princess. I want you to take especially good care of her.'"

Clearly **Lucy** knows that in the scheme of things this little conversation is insignificant, but said to her it was symbolic of something more. "I feel like I am being noticed again instead of just fading into the woodwork".

> "We face a world where 'lookism' is one of the most pervasive but denied prejudices. People like to believe that looks don't matter. But every marketing executive knows that packaging and image are as important as the product, if not more so. We treat appearance not just as a source of pleasure or shame but as a source of information." **7**

It makes us feel good to be noticed by men, but I wanted to know if increased visibility ever led to life altering events. When I posed this question to **Denise**, she first spoke about her client, **Joyce**, a woman who had once been so beautiful that she had won a national beauty contest. "But by age fifty-three, she felt devastated by her loss of good looks, felt anonymous and overlooked." After her cosmetic surgery **Joyce** joined match.com. and got responses from seventy-five men, including the plastic surgeon who had done her surgery; but even he did not recognize her. She didn't respond to him, but experienced so many more social opportunities that she speaks about her refreshed appearance as a "social rebirth" for her.

Denise mentioned that for those who want to take advantage of the Internet, a technology that has become such a popular vehicle for placing personal ads, appearance becomes more important than ever before.

> "Your face is going to be right out there, the first thing viewers see when they scan the screen. They will pass right by you if they aren't attracted to your face, no matter how many wonderful virtues you possess. We are living in such a busy world that

sometimes that first impression is the only opportunity we get to open a door for ourselves."

The happiest story Denise shared was about **Elizabeth**, a woman who adopted a baby girl at age forty-six and had a facelift several years later. At age fifty-four she became widowed, but then fell in love with a pilot four years after her husband's death. She told Denise: "I act silly now, and am having such fun. Believe me, none of this would have happened with my old, haggard face". Even her teenage daughter has noticed and commented: "Mom, I never knew old people could giggle and have so much."

Studies have repeatedly documented different aspects to preferential treatment for physically attractive people. No discussion on this topic would be complete without reference to Dr. Nancy Etcoff's pioneering work. Here are the results of two studies she details in her book, *Survival of the Prettiest*: **8**

In this first study, psychologists set up a situation in which men and women who had never met were instructed to engage in ten minute phone conversations. Each man was given a photograph of the woman with whom he was supposed to be talking. Although some photos revealed beautiful women and others, very unattractive ones, in fact each man would be talking to the same woman.

Each time a man was speaking to a woman he perceived as beautiful, he tried harder to be charming, bolder, sexier and wittier. Interestingly, in each instance her conversations became more animated and confidant, bolder and sexier when she felt she was perceived as attractive. **9**

In the second study, people were given photographs of pre and post-operative cosmetic surgery patients and in each case were asked to make judgments about their personalities and their effectiveness as marriage partners. The post-operative photo group received consistently higher evaluation scores for having desirable personalities, being happier and being better potential marriage partners. **10**

Not only did the physically attractive people in these studies receive preferential treatment, but that special treatment helped shape their consequent behaviors and self-perceptions. Here we see that self-fulfilling prophecy at work once again. The "Frankenstein perspective" tells us that the way the world sees us is what we become.

This last story has nothing to do with improved careers, bestowed favors or more overt interest from men. It is about how our legal system favors the physically attractive.

> "Law enforcement officials, juries and judges don't just judge the current circumstances and the person's past behavior but they take a look and think: Could she have done that? The effect is particularly strong for attractive females." **11**

When I asked **Gail**, the professional singer you first met in Chapter 1, *Cosmetic Surgery, The Aphrodisiac Effect,* if she has noted any incidences of preferential treatment, she talked about one experience that happened about six months after her cosmetic surgery.

She was on her way to a rehearsal when she was suddenly overcome by stomach sickness. She parked her car in a nearby available spot and rushed into the lady's room in an adjacent restaurant.

"I didn't notice that I had parked in a *No Standing* zone, but when I returned to my car, I discovered a ticket with a $75 fine on my windshield. I wrote a letter of explanation and was asked to appear in court. I dressed very carefully for that court appearance. My hair, my make-up, my clothes . . My neighbor reinforced my good feelings as I was about to leave. 'You look so great. I'll bet that if you have a male judge, he's going to rescind that fine.' "

Gail continued her story about how she had to sit through twenty some cases before it was her turn. She said she listened to many convincing arguments, but the judge was really strict and didn't dismiss a single case and the officer who had written all their tickets was even worse - mean and argumentative with each of them.

"When my turn finally came, I spoke softly, looked the judge in the eye and made my case. I could tell from his expression that he was definitely impressed, and as much as we hate to admit that physical appearance could influence the outcome of a case, I know in my heart that it did. He smiled at me and said: 'This was clearly an emergency situation. I dismiss this case.'"

Gail said she thanked him and turned to leave, but half way down the steps, heard a male voice calling after her.

"It was the same arrogant officer, but now he was sweet as sugar. First he engaged me in conversation as he followed me to my car. He inquired if I had gotten the flu, if this had ever happened to me before, stuff like that. We had a little more friendly conversation, I thanked him for his understanding, then he opened my car door to help me enter and we said good night."

Gail was aware of other people in that courtroom who deserved to have their cases dismissed that night and felt a bit guilty about how she got that advantage. "Appearance matters, even in legal matters", she said.

When I asked Gail if she thought there were other factors that might have influenced the outcome of her case, she hesitated before answering: "My renewed appearance gave me a feeling of confidence. I know that helped me present my argument well."

What ever happened to the notion that beauty is only skin deep? At one time a person's education, family background and character were what counted most; but in today's fast paced world, first impressions often take precedence. As we noted earlier, today the first impression we make on others is often the only opportunity we get to make things happen for ourselves, socially and in the workplace.

And yet, I can think of many exceptions - people who achieved greatness despite unexceptional physical presence. Israel's former prime minister, Golda Mier and former Secretary of State, Madeline Albright, were never noted for their beauty, but achieved greatness due to their intelligence, commitment, courage and strong negotiating skills. Even in the field of entertainment, where beauty is most often revered; many times talent and hard work reap greater rewards. Fantasia didn't win the American Idol 2004 title based on her looks. It was her talent that wooed young Americans, who showed their appreciation for her vocal style by casting the majority of those final 65,000 votes in her direction.

I can report to you from my experiences as an educator that at the beginning of each school year, children assigned to one young, pretty teacher reacted with special glee while those assigned to another teacher on that grade level appeared far less enthused. But as each school year wore on, it was the wrinkled, overweight teacher who became everyone's favorite. Why? She created an atmosphere in which children felt valued and admired. She taught them the most powerful lesson of their lives: to believe in themselves.

This physical attractiveness stereotype does have its limitations. It seems strongest when people are judged for immediacy or for social factors, especially those involving the opposite sex. But other virtues such as integrity, competence, intelligence, talent, humor, loyalty, nurturance, concern for others and sensitivity to their needs . . . become recognizable with increased associations. Friends, colleagues and family members have that opportunity to get to know us in more than a surface way. As they share experiences, discover common interests and thoughts; relate to our conversations, the stereotype is likely to lessen or virtually disappear.

I like to think that acts of human kindness, a good sense of humor, being an interesting and interested human being, caring about others, excelling in your life's work . . . still count in our world. I hope I'm not being overly naïve to think that they do.

When your inner beauty matches your outer beauty, you've really got it made!

Helpful Resources

See also the following end-of-book helpful resources pertinent to information found in this chapter.

 CD Part B: Test Your Self-Esteem

Appendix 8: Personal Profiles
(More about the people whose
names appear in this chapter)

Footnotes

1. Cash TF. and Pruzinsky T. eds. Body Image: A Handbook of Theory, Research and Clinical Practice. New York. Guilford Press. (2002): 37.

2. Langlois JH. Ritter LA. Roggman LA. and Vaughan LS. "Facial diversity and facial preferences for attractive faces." Developmental Psychology. 27 (1991): 79-84.

3. Langlois JH. Roggman LA. Casey RJ. Ritter LA. Reiser-Danner A. and Jenkins VY. "Infant preferences for attractive faces: rudiments of a stereotype." Developmental Psychology. 23. (1987): 363-369.

4. Dion KK. and Berscheid E. "Physical attractiveness and peer perception among children." Sociometry. 37. (1974): 1-12.

5. Sarwer DB. and Magee L. "Physical Appearance and Society". In. Psychological Aspects of Reconstructive and Cosmetic Plastic Surgery: Clinical, Empirical and Ethical Perspectives. Lippincott, Williams and Wilkens (Sept. 2005)).

6. Garner D. "The body image survey." Psychology Today. 30.1 (Feb. 97): 30(18).

7. Etcoff N. Survival of the Prettiest -The Science of Beauty. Doubleday (1999): 39..

8. Etcoff N. Survival of the Prettiest -The Science of Beauty. Doubleday (1999): 38.

9. Snyder ED. Tanke and Berscheid E. "Social perception and interpersonal behavior: on the self-fulfilling nature of social stereotypes." Journal of Personality and Social Psychology. 35 (1977): 656-666.

10. Cunningham MR. "Measuring the physical in physical attractiveness: quasi experiments on the sociobiology of female facial beauty". Journal of Personality and Social Psychology. 50.(1986): 925-935.

11. Etcoff N. Survival of the Prettiest -The Science of Beauty. Doubleday (1999): 49.

Chapter 5: Utter Humiliation

The Short Story:

The day I lost my dignity

"Humiliation: Reduction of one's self-respect or dignity"

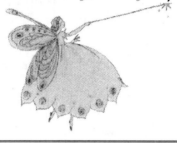

"It has been my pleasure to have worked with Lois in many capacities. Such a fine lady, and she is that in every sense of the word too! Imagine – a supremely professional teacher and a lady – all in one package. This is not too easy to replace – I would wager impossible."

"You are an inspiration! A lady – always – in the truest sense of the word. An enlightened educator, creative and a sensitive, supportive colleague besides!"

I found the above two messages written in my retirement album, the first from a building principal, the second from a Special Education teacher. Funny how often the word 'lady' appeared in words written and spoken to me that evening. For that matter, throughout my lifetime.

This chapter tells a different story. It's the story of the day I blew my cover – shed my ladylike demeanor. It's the day I felt all those lessons instilled from childhood slip out into the wind. This is how it began.

In the weeks following my surgery I had begun to develop a questionnaire for cosmetic surgery patients. I wanted to explore some rather straightforward topics as:

How did other women go about selecting their plastic surgeons? What were some of the most common motivations for plastic surgery? How did other women find recovery in terms of discomfort and time lost from their lives?

I thought it would be interesting to get answers to these questions and more, to look at the collective experiences of many women who had undergone cosmetic surgery. But then those other things began to happen, those emotionally charged feelings of inordinate happiness that made me feel changed in at first inexplicable ways.

My physical healing had gone so well – quickly, easily, with only mild discomfort after the first few days. But emotionally I needed to readjust. No one had ever told me that there would be an emotional component to this process. I wasn't prepared for it – didn't anticipate any of it – especially the part that happened next.

My fantasy life went into high gear with my plastic surgeon always the protagonist to my creations. But he no longer appeared in his surgical scrubs or one of his finely tailored suits. There he was in his shiny silver gym shorts, leaping hurdles of nearly insurmountable heights as he sprinted forward. I was always right there at the finish line.

And that was how my fantasies began. They became more inventive from that point forward.

I had heard my psychologist friends from work speak of transference, so at least I knew this was a common phenomenon - something patients frequently felt toward their therapists. I guessed, correctly, that it was probably the same thing operating here, but somehow this knowledge gave me little comfort. Nonetheless I plunged forward and added several new questions to my ever expanding repertoire of questionnaire topics, including the following intimate probe:

Question #37. Which statement best describes your feelings toward you plastic surgeon?
Here are the choices I presented:

> **a)** I maintained a purely professional, non-emotional relationship with my plastic surgeon.
> **b)** I felt warmed by how much s/he cared about me as a human being, not just a patient.
> **c)** I found my plastic surgeon increasingly attractive with each visit.
> **d)** Thinking about my plastic surgeon provided me with a rich source of sensual fantasies which I found unsettling.
> **e)** Thinking about my plastic surgeon provided me with a rich source of sensual fantasies which I enjoyed.
> **f)** I might act on my impulses if I had a chance.
> **g)** I have in fact acted on my impulses.

I fit right into category **d)**. I was feeling unglued. To make matters worse, in two days I had a scheduled meeting with Dr. K…. to review the contents of this questionnaire. He had generously offered to read and add his input to my book and had been doing so on an ongoing basis. How was I ever going to face him now?

Just keep your composure, I told myself as I neared his office door. *Present all your questions professionally - with detachment – and you will be fine.* I continued to prep myself as I waited for his arrival in the small room where I was now seated. And that's how I began, professionally, with outward composure.

I made it through all the questions on sensuality and sexuality without a hitch. I don't think I ever blushed. I didn't detect any break in my voice. But as I neared question #37, my heart began to race, my hands turned to ice. I just didn't think I was going to be able to hold it together for question #37.

And then I had a sudden epiphany:
Surely Dr. K.... has heard this hundreds of times before. This must even be part of every plastic surgeon's medical school training – a course listed in the catalogues as Transference 207. If only I could manage to tell him what was troubling me, he would be able to help me through it. So I took a deep breath and began. The conversation, to the best of my recollection, went something like this:

"Okay, now for question #37. This one is going to be very uncomfortable for me to talk about. It has to do with transference." As I hand him this page of the questionnaire I say: "You see, this has become an issue for me."

"Oh, I see", says Dr. K.... in his most dignified manner, as he begins to read question #37.

I feel a need to fill the dead air space so I continue.

> "You know, I consider myself pretty well grounded, pretty stable, so I figure if this is happening to me, if I'm feeling some of these feelings, it must have happened with some of your other patients who are more extreme, some who even have crossed over that line."

He nods his head in agreement as he quietly, almost imperceptibly, leans forward and nudges the door that separates us from the hallway a bit further ajar.

Oh, good lord, he must think I'm about to pounce, I think to myself. I hasten to reassure him and dig my hole a few feet deeper.

> "Dr. K…., you'll never have to worry about me acting on my impulses. My dignity is far too important to me. I mean, you'll never need to call a nurse into the room with us. I just would never allow myself to do anything inappropriate."

I hear all these words come tumbling from my mouth, but somehow can't fathom the idea that I am the one uttering them. There must be a ventriloquist in this room.

I have now passed beyond sheer embarrassment to utter humiliation.

He maintains a compassionate, accepting tone as he tells me he always likes to get to know the patients with whom he works. Somehow he manages to interweave into this conversation a story about one husband's verbal abuse toward his wife by disparaging her acne scarred skin. (I no longer recall how this connected with the rest of our conversation, but it seemed relevant at the time.) He offers to publicize my questionnaire in his next newsletter, but requests that I first remove question #37. I agree. I'm too rattled to focus on anything – even the generosity of his offer. I can only focus on my feelings of despair.

"This has been a very difficult conversation for me.", I manage to say.

He smiles sympathetically. I know he would help me if he could. He just never took that course, Transference 207, in medical school. Now I realize it probably doesn't exist. I leave convinced he thinks I'm a putrid degenerate.

The second I arrive home I dart to my bathroom medicine cabinet and gulp down two Excedrin. I feel about two inches tall. How could I have been so foolish? Why did I assume that just because he was a talented plastic surgeon, he would know the answers to such psychologically based questions? What I needed at that moment was someone who was psychologically savvy – someone who could help me through this creeping anxiety. I reached for the phone to call a former colleague.

Lorraine Schles-Esposito and I worked together on many hundreds of cases before the Committee of Special Education. I think of her not just as a trusted friend, but as a skilled psychologist, perceptive observer and clever problem solver. I dialed her number. After a few preliminary words I said: "Lorraine, I really need to talk to you – quickly." We met in a local diner the following afternoon.

In less than two minutes I brought her up to speed and then plunged forward.

> "Lorraine, I need you to tell me everything you know about transference. This has hit me so hard and I just can't control it. I feel like I'm coming unglued. Does this mean that I have all kinds of suppressed feelings that I've never dealt with?"

> "No, that's a very Freudian view", she says. " I don't see it that way at all. Transference happens when one person views another as being instrumental in affecting change within him or herself. So the question you want to explore is this. What changes do you feel within yourself since your surgery?"

I gave Lorraine a brief summary of how cosmetic surgery had changed the way I feel about myself, within myself. I told her about all the little self-improvement projects I had initiated after my surgery (weight loss, exercises, change of hair style, skin care, etc.).

"At first I thought this was all about vanity, and I didn't even *like* myself for feeling so good about such superficial things. Then one day it struck me that it wasn't so much how I looked that was making me feel so happy, it was the feeling of femininity, the feeling of sexuality that was empowering me. Then those feelings helped me look at other aspects of my life more openly, more assertively."

Lorraine, never for a loss of words, continued.

"You know, when I first met you, all I saw was this very professional person, impeccably dressed, refined and capable, but fairly reserved. Then, when I got to know you better, I discovered a whole different person there. Just the way you viewed things, not at all provincial, quite open minded. Sometimes you'd come out with some really funny, uninhibited responses. I've learned that I can tell a lot about a person by their humor. I guess I was surprised to find such a sensual person under that façade."

"Oh, my lord, I never think of myself that way," I tell her.

"Really? That could be a little self-denial on your part. But it stands to reason. You project such a ladylike image that that's the way most people will relate to you. Generally a person needs to project a sensual image to get that kind of feedback from others. My guess is that you probably had a very proper upbringing."

"Oh, that's for sure! Dance classes with white gloves – always a curtsy to your partner. Oh, brother, did I ever feel those white gloves slip off my hands and land with a thud, right in front of Dr. K..... And then, all those years at Friends Academy, each Wednesday we would gather together at the Quaker meeting

61

house, sit on those hard wooden benches and think noble thoughts. Where were all my noble thoughts yesterday? They really abandoned me when I needed them most.'

"As for sex, that's a word that was hardly mentioned in my family. Or if it was, I certainly never got the impression that this was supposed to be a pleasurable activity for women. I had to figure that one out for myself! But it took me a long time. When I was fifteen, even sixteen, I would hear my campmates say things like: 'Oh, above the waist is alright'. But not me – it was more like 'above the neck' for me.

I never lacked for dates because I was reasonably attractive, but more than that, I was enthusiastic. I was shy, but I knew how to have a good time. I loved to dance, play tennis, swim, go biking. And then when I enrolled at Barnard, I fell in love with all the museums, theatre. It opened up new worlds for me. But as soon as a guy would move in, get a little physical, I was out of there. I'd tell my roommate, 'I thought he was such a nice guy, but what a pig he turned out to be.' That didn't change much for me until I met Ken. Then trust me, it changed in a hurry!

Can you believe that Ken has been the sum of most of my lifetime sexual experiences? I know by today's standards I'm absolutely archaic."

"Lois, don't you see? That's just why this experience has been so hard for you to handle. We were brought up during a time when there were so many imposed inhibitions. Today it's different. Today most young people are much more relaxed in their attitudes."

I realize that Lorraine and I have now spent over an hour and a half, dipping crackers in our bowls of pea soup, talking and listening in turn. It felt good to leave some of that tension behind.

"Let's get back to transference", I say, bringing us back to my immediate topic of concern. "I want to be sure I understand this in terms of myself. Are you saying that cosmetic surgery was a catalyst for me – an event that changed the way I feel about myself, changed things that I see as positives within my life?"

"That's right. And to take it one step further, you see your surgeon as that agent of change. You feel so appreciative of what he's done for you. Not just because he made you look younger, but because of the inner changes your surgery has evoked. That's really what it's all about."

"Everything you say makes perfect sense to me, and I'm sure that's a big part of what's happening here. But I think there is something else. Something I can't quite put my finger on. It has to do with when a man looks at you, your physical being, and makes you feel like in his eyes you are an attractive woman. This person literally has transformed you, made you suddenly feel so wonderful about yourself. It reminds me of the way I felt when Ken and I first fell in love. He would look at me with such obvious pleasure. That was such a magical time – to feel absolutely adored by a man whom I saw as such a special person."

"But love is different, Lois. A surgeon doesn't do cosmetic surgery for love. He does it for other reasons – for aesthetics, for money, maybe because he knows he's a really skilled plastic surgeon and his results continually reinforce that feel-good feeling within himself. I'm not sure about this other part. You might just have to wait until you get a chance to speak with other women. See what they have to say. You are really exploring some untapped territory here. If you can get women to open up, share their feelings, it should be enlightening, to say the least."

I had been on overload, but now I felt a bit easier. "Oh Lorraine, thank you, you've really helped me today. I feel so much better, but also pretty stupid."

"Well, you shouldn't. Most women wouldn't even admit to themselves the things you said to your surgeon. My guess is that many women *show* their plastic surgeons how they feel by their behavior, by sexual overture, but I doubt that many speak so openly about their feelings. Your doctor may not even have made the connection between your words and outward displays of sexuality he probably gets from other patients. You're just a bit stunned to realize that even a stable, intelligent, happily married woman can be subject to such an emotional event. I think what you did was very courageous."

"This is what you call courage?" I say. "Do you realize that I actually *told* this agent-of-change that he was enriching my fantasy life? I can't believe I said all that. He must think I'm either the village idiot or some kind of a deviant."

"Oh, don't worry about it", she said. "You probably put a buzz on him for the rest of the week. He's human too you know."

Six Tips for Cosmetic Surgery Patients

If you are a woman who has recently undergone cosmetic surgery, and find yourself increasingly attracted to your plastic surgeon, I offer you a few words of wisdom from the trenches of one who has been there.

1. Know that transference - a feeling of sexual attraction - is a phenomenon that you may experience toward your plastic surgeon. If it happens to you, don't freak out. Understand it.

2. Have the good sense to keep your feelings to yourself. Don't share them with your plastic surgeon unless you enjoy feeling two inches tall. Don't share them with your husband or significant other. I did and when Ken asked, "What exactly is transference?" I knew I was in trouble. (Apparently they don't offer the course Transference 207 at Yale Law School either.)

3. Try to uncover the reason this is happening to you. Ask yourself, "How do I feel differently about myself since my cosmetic surgery?" Try to get below the surface to the core of your personal transitions. But be gentle with yourself. Raw emotions can be hard to handle.

4. Keep in mind that it is your plastic surgeon's talent and skill that have made you feel like a more desirable woman. He is probably genuinely happy he has been able to bring you such joy. His compliments are simply his way of expressing his pleasure in aesthetics, his feeling of creating more beauty in this world. This is his life's work. It is not his life's work to become personally involved with any of his patients. Remember, when you leave his examining room, another woman enters.

5. If you can't work through your feelings on your own and they continue to trouble you, it may be time for you to consider some professional advice.

6. If you don't need to work this through, if you're enjoying your fantasies, what the heck, have a wonderful journey! Write them down and put them away in a safe place or share them with your best friend. She'll probably enjoy them too.

Read this chapter several times. You might just find glimmers of yourself hidden within these pages.

Six Tips for Plastic Surgeons

Now, if you are a plastic surgeon who is confronted by a patient such as me, here are some tips for you:

1. Know that transference, a feeling of sexual attraction toward one's plastic surgeon, is a phenomenon that might occur. Understand that it is not your baby blue eyes or scintillating personality that sends her home all aquiver. It's more a matter of how you made her feel about herself. Understand the dynamics and you will be better able to handle these situations as they arise.

And when it happens, pat yourself on the back for your skill as a surgeon, not for your sexual magnetism.

2. If you are a plastic surgeon who is confronted by a patient such as me, first you need to decide for yourself if you want to have any dialogue on this topic. (Only you know your own comfort level.) If you feel uncomfortable, you will unknowingly communicate those feelings and compound the problem. If you prefer to avoid a big discussion, you might say something like this:

> "Yes, I know this is a common feeling women develop toward their plastic surgeons, but it's a little beyond my area of expertise. If you think you would like to talk this through a little more, why don't you set up a time to talk with ___ ."

Select one of your nurses whom you know would be willing and capable of addressing this issue. Be sure she has some names available for psychological referrals if it appears advisable.

3. If you choose to respond, do so with care. Your patient is probably at her most vulnerable and could easily misinterpret your words as either rejection or encouragement. You might simply say:

> "I'm not a psychologist, but I know this usually happens because of other feelings of change that a person can experience following cosmetic surgery."

Know that your exact words will matter far less than your ability to convey an accepting tone and cordial manner.

4. Maintain your professionalism. Do not take advantage of an all too human situation. If you think this is an unnecessary warning, please read the next chapter carefully. Furthermore, you are human too, and as such can be subject to feelings of counter transference.

5. Whether you choose to respond directly or not, you now have a resource to offer. You can say:

> "I know of one woman who experienced some of the very same feelings you are feeling right now and wrote about them in her book: *Sex, Lies and Cosmetic Surgery*. I think you'll really enjoy it and at the same time find it helpful. She has a lighthearted approach, writes with a lot of humor, but offers wonderful insights."

I hope you truly feel that way; but even if you don't, I won't object if you say it anyway.

6. This final tip comes from **Lorraine**:

> "I think it would be just wonderful if something could be added to each surgeon's pre-care surgery packet to start the patient's thought process in the right direction. Something that shares the fact that people can experience a resurgence of difficult-to-explain feelings following cosmetic surgery - that this is not uncommon during the post surgery adjustment process, is usually very positive, but might take some

time to sort through. That would kind of open the door for patients to allow themselves to face their feelings, even speak about them if they felt a need."

Helpful Resources

See also the following end-of-book helpful resources pertinent to information found in this chapter.

☼ **Appendix 8: Personal Profiles**
   (More about the people whose
   names appear in this chapter)

Chapter 6: You Might Fall in Love With Your Plastic Surgeon

The Short Story:
Patients and professionals speak out about amorous feelings toward their plastic surgeons

"Amorous: Full of love"

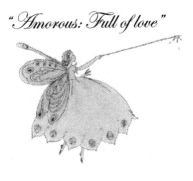

Did other women experience similar feelings toward their plastic surgeons? I needed confirmation, but found none in the responses women provided on their cosmetic surgery questionnaire forms.

Many, including **'Realtor'**, **Hartley**, **'Snowbird'**, **'Beauty Queen'**, **'Makeover'** and **'Jockette'** selected **a)** *I maintained a purely professional, non-emotional relationship with my plastic surgeon.* **Hope** and **'Small'** selected **b)** *I felt warmed by how much he cared about me as a human being – not just as a patient.* **'Sunshine'** wrote: *None – he's just a sweetheart who is funny, kind and caring.* Then she added her own postscript: *Not the way I felt about my obstetrician, where I did experience lots of those kind of feelings.*

As I began to investigate further, I discovered a brief description, written by journalist Helen Bransford, where she spoke about being afflicted with 'PAP (Physician Appreciation Phase)' following her own facelift. She described those feelings as being as powerful as any hormone one is likely to have ever known, comparable to that first kiss, and cautioned women to exercise restraint. **1**

I searched for more evidence and finally, within a Vogue Magazine article, uncovered this explanation by Dr. David Sarwer, Associate Professor of Psychology at the University of Pennsylvania School of Medicine:

> "Working with any health professional can be a very intimate experience. They're physically close to us, and they see us when we're most vulnerable.'

> Then, in speaking about the cosmetic surgery patient, he continued: "Patients attribute their good feelings to the doctor, when in fact, it's the change in their appearance that has made them feel better. The patient may confuse the positive feelings with romantic love. The relationship with the cosmetic surgeon is different than with other doctors, because it's related to beauty and appearance, which are associated with romance and sexuality." **2**

I was a perfect match for Dr. Sarwer's analysis.

When I asked **Denise** what she knew about transference, she passed my question along to a plastic surgery nurse and personal friend of hers. Her friend laughed as she told Denise that right after the new privacy regulations went into effect, a patient she called **Lily** whispered to her: "I think he has a crush on me. Today he opened the door to the waiting room and called out: 'L.Z., you're next. He never called me by my initials before." The nurse had to explain that as part of the new privacy regulations, doctors had been advised to no longer announce any patient's name in front of other patients.

I wanted more data. To that end I next interviewed a Manhattan based cosmetic surgery nurse/esthetician whose client base includes the patients of several prominent plastic surgeons. Because she requested anonymity, I refer to her as **Beauty** in the verbatim transcript that follows:

LWS: "From your vantage point, do you think women often develop feelings of sexual attraction toward their plastic surgeons?"

Beauty: "Oh, yes. It's very common."

LWS: "Then I'd like to ask you two questions: 'What do you observe that makes you say that?' and 'When do you think that attraction usually starts?' "

Beauty: "I often notice this right after surgery. A woman is just coming out of anesthesia and I'll hear her say, 'Oh, I love you', to her surgeon. This is something she does when her defenses are down, when she's not able to monitor her words and not consciously aware of what she is saying. But notice, she doesn't say, 'I love you, Harry' or 'I love you Jim'. She isn't reaching out to her husband. She is definitely speaking to her surgeon. She doesn't remember any of this later on, but I've heard it many times."

LWS: "How do the surgeons respond?"

Beauty: "Oh, usually they do something gentle like touch the woman's arm, say something to comfort her, to sooth her at that moment. It means nothing more."

LWS: "What about later on, when women are in the process of healing? Are you aware of this attraction then too? If so, how do they show it?"

Beauty: "Well, first of all, it's the way some women dress when they come for follow-up visits. They dress provocatively. I've seen more than one woman come to her post-surgery appointments in underwear or blouse so sheer that she might as well have worn a transparent negligee. I've also seen women back their plastic surgeons into a corner, actually brush their breasts up against his arm or side."

LWS: "On one level, I'm surprised by such aggression, but on another level, I think it's almost predictable. Are you aware of any other ways those feelings come through?"

Beauty: "Sure. Don't forget I'm the one who sees many of these women on a regular basis long after their surgeries. Some women are very subtle. They will ask me questions about their surgeon's personal life: *How old is he? Is he married? What does his wife look like?* Others will tell me exactly how they feel. They lie on my table in a dimly lit room with their eyes closed. They just relax and then sometimes they talk to me about those things."

LWS: "Do they ever talk about their own emotional responses to these sexual feelings?"

Beauty: "Some women feel embarrassed. Others openly pursue them. They will say things like, 'Last time we met, I think we really made a connection.' I've known of times when they've actually stalked a doctor – hung out outside his office building or in the parking garage where he keeps his car. Women can be very inventive, do a lot of detective work in order to find all kinds of methods to approach their plastic surgeons in unexpected places and ways."

LWS: "How do the surgeons respond to this?"

Beauty: "Some buy into it. It inflates their egos – gives them a God like persona. Others are just more focused on their work and don't really pay much attention to these behaviors."

Me: "You know, before my surgery, if anyone had ever told me I would get caught up in this, I would have said, 'You've got to be out of your mind!' And yet I did. Why do you think this is so common?"

Beauty: "I think it is all about confirming your feminine side - confirming you as a sexual human being."

LWS: "It seems to me it must be very difficult to be the wife of a plastic surgeon. I personally would hate living with the knowledge that other women are actively pursuing my husband, and suspect that this could take a real toll on a marriage."

Beauty: "Oh, I totally agree. I think it's a hard role for those wives to play."

In her Vogue article, Elizabeth Hayt wrote about patients' crushes on their plastic surgeons and shared some thoughts from one surgeon's wife, who discussed this not infrequent situation. Upon being introduced to one of her husband's patients, she occasionally hears words such as: "Oh, so you are Dr. H . . .'s wife. I LOVE him." The surgeon's wife claims to never know the right response. Should she admire the patient's good taste or say what she really feels: "I was there first."? **3**

I asked **Nicole**, the creator and owner of the most active Internet Breast Augmentation site, if women ever speak to her about feelings of attraction toward their surgeons. Although this wasn't the case for her as her surgeon was much older than she and more like a father figure, she said she has seen many such postings on this topic on her discussion boards.

> "Women look and feel so wonderful after surgery and are filled with such gratitude toward the person who helped them feel that way. That feeling can spill over into a romantic notion about the surgeon."

Judy, the interior designer who had reconstructive surgery, spoke about her growing feelings of attraction toward her reconstructive surgeon. "At first I was hesitant about him even touching me. I thought he was so insensitive." **Judy** continued by explaining that before surgery, he had come into the room and just said: 'Take your top off and let me photograph you.' She felt such a lack of respect and only went along with him because she held her breast surgeon, who had recommended him, in such high regard and trusted her judgment.

But in time, this reconstructive surgeon won **Judy's** heart and became "one of the warmest, most responsive doctors I have ever known." Although she was able to speak about her strong attraction toward her surgeon during that six week period of aftercare without a hint of discomfort, **Zena** was clearly embarrassed and needed reassurances before she shared her story:

> "Even before my facelift I was beginning to feel some attraction toward my plastic surgeon. But in the weeks afterwards, those feelings began to explode – really get out of control. Several months after my facelift, I told my surgeon that I thought I might like to have a breast lift. Do you know why? I knew he would have to examine me, and I wanted him to touch me, to put his hands on my body. That's how crazy I was. And you know what? It felt really good."

Even **Gail**, the soft spoken, professional singer who preferred quiet, fireside evenings with her husband, had an experience to share. "I became totally obsessed with thoughts about my plastic surgeon. I'd get emotional and somewhat tingly each time I thought about seeing him again. I had this one fantasy thing that I kept replaying in my head, but I'd just be too embarrassed to tell you."

Usually the flirtatious feelings that surface are harmless and eventually evaporate, but in the next two cases, they created emotional havoc. **Amy** described her experience as "beyond horrible" and "one of the most embarrassing episodes of my life."

As background, she explained that her plastic surgeon has privileges at the same hospital as her physician husband who recommended him:

> "I never felt any particular attraction for this man before he became my plastic surgeon, but then those feelings grew so intense that I barely could think of anyone but him. On one of my follow-up appointments, as I spoke to him, tears began to flow. When he asked what was troubling me, I blurted out: 'I love you and want to leave my husband so that I can be free to marry you.'
>
> He asked me to set up another appointment at the end of that day so that he could talk to me and my husband together. He recommended a psychiatrist so that we could consider medication. Thank G-- they put me an anti-depressant. Afterwards I felt so horrible – I just hated myself for what I had done."

Julie's experience was even more traumatic. At age thirty-two she suddenly became widowed, left with two small children to raise on her own. Ten years after her husband's death, one of her friends convinced her to get her eyes done. "She told me it would give me both a psychological and cosmetic lift and recommended me to her surgeon." **Julie** liked him right away, mostly because he seemed to be a good listener and empathetic and gave her lots of compliments. But after surgery, something else began to happen:

> "I could feel myself becoming attracted to him – leaning in toward him when we talked, dressing up for him when I came for my follow-up visits. Then one day we just ended up in an embrace right there in

one of his examining rooms. Bells went off. I truly thought I had fallen in love with this man."

She let nature take its course, and they began having late afternoon trysts.

Julie was ecstatic. Life had begun again and she felt like she had found that perfect man - until he started giving excuses for why they couldn't meet. Somehow she became suspicious, did a little investigative work and discovered that he was seeing another one of his patients. After her, there was a third. Apparently this was a regular pattern for him. "Many years have passed, but I still see this as the most difficult experience of my life – even more painful than becoming a widow. Eventually he was brought up on charges , but then I lost track of what happened to him.

Julie ended our conversation with the words:

> "Believe me, I'm not faulting plastic surgeons, I know that most of them are highly respectable, but there are a few bad apples in every profession. I've never told this to anyone before, but I think a woman is especially vulnerable after cosmetic surgery, feeling more attractive and ready to have those feelings confirmed. That's why I'm telling you my story. I want you to caution your readers to be aware, to not allow themselves to get carried away."

I returned to **Denise** to ask if she had anything further to add.

> "In a patient/doctor relationship, social interactions should be verboten on any level. If a client tells me she is attracted to her surgeon, I quickly caution her not to waste her time, at least while she is currently his patient."

Denise knows that doctors are sometimes confronted with

these situations and although she didn't think a course existed such as Patients 101, she supposed the topic might come up at some of their plastic surgery meetings.

She also knows most doctors take common sense precautions such as to always have a nurse present in the examining room for any form of body exam, to never unnecessarily touch a woman – even her shoulder or elbow - as they escort her to an examining room, and to only touch the parts of her body necessary for the examination, nothing more.

I asked her if she could describe a scenario of how she supposed a plastic surgeon would handle the persistent patient. Here is her description:

> "Picture a younger woman who keeps making follow-up appointments with her surgeon. She wears sexy underwear, provocative clothing and strong perfume each time she sees him. Perhaps she gives him a gift or gets a little touchy feely. When she returns once again for another extra visit, he might say something like: 'Mrs. T. What is the problem? It's ninety days since your surgery. I will have to begin to charge you for any further visits.'

> "She might even begin to stalk him, find out the location of the gym where he works out or the night when he generally goes to the opera and just happen to arrive in time to accidentally-on-purpose bump into him. This behavior calls for severe measures. He might send her a certified letter saying that he has dismissed her as a patient and advise her to go to the emergency room if she has further problems, but this would be most unlikely so many months after surgery."

Several years after my surgery and many months after I thought I had completed my manuscript, I received a phone call from a woman named **Betsy.** She was considering cosmetic surgery, had heard that I was writing a book and had done considerable research, and wondered if I would be willing to talk with her. We spoke on the phone that day, but it wasn't until after she had gone to her third consultation that we actually met. Then we talked about the three surgeons with whom she had consulted and her impressions of each of them. Her observations were astute and professional, not personal.

But when we met again just ten days after her surgery, she enthused about her surgeon of choice.

> "I never noticed how handsome he is. And he's so charming as well! I must have been going on and on about him to the man I recently began dating, because he said, 'You certainly are taken with him', but clearly he wasn't enjoying this conversation."

I couldn't resist a word of motherly advice. "Be careful, **Betsy**", I cautioned. "I have a chapter in my book entitled *You Might Fall in Love with Your Plastic Surgeon.*" Her eyes grew wide with astonishment, but I just smiled knowingly.

Helpful Resources

See also the following end-of-book helpful resources pertinent to information found in this chapter.

🔔 **Appendix 8: Personal Profiles**
   (More about the people whose names appear in this chapter)

🔔 **Appendix 9: Additional Stories for Chapter 6**

Footnotes

1. Bransford H. <u>Welcome to Your Facelift</u>. Doubleday. 1997. Main Street Books, 1998. 144.

2. Sarwer DB. In. <u>Vogue Magazine.</u> (March 2000): 422.

3. Hayt E. "Dr. Strangelove". <u>Vogue Magazine.</u> (March 2000): 427.

The Short Story:
Motivations and catalysts to
cosmetic surgery

"Motivation: A stimulus or influence"
"Catalyst: An agent that provides significant change"

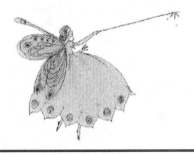

My Story: Stirrings of Discontent

I accepted my school district's 'first eligible' retirement offer
in exchange for full medical benefits. I had loved my work,
but felt ready to sprout my wings, pursue some other
interests, challenge myself anew.

On the evening of my retirement party, I listened to the
Superintendent of Schools begin her farewell address to me
- with a reading from a book of Politically Correct Fairy
Tales:

*Long, long ago there lived a person of better than average
attractiveness . . .*

Her reading struck me as a rather unusual introduction to a
farewell address, but I had to admit that her words were a
fairly accurate reflection of my private self-image. I still felt

basically good about the way I looked – not drop dead gorgeous, but attractive enough to keep me feeling confident about my appearance.

She continued:

As the years passed, Rosamond grew into an intelligent, compassionate, and self-actualized wommon.

This, too, seemed an apt summation of my private self-image. I was never a woman who defined herself by her physical presence. Don't get me wrong. I liked looking good, feeling attractive; but I was far less caught up in the trappings of cosmetics, fashion and jewelry than most. I looked upon my accomplishments as the essence of me – a solid marriage, two wonderful sons, strong professional contributions, good friends. These were the ultimate yardsticks to my self-worth.

After retirement, this woman of reasonable intelligence, 'better-than-average attractiveness' and eagerness to explore new vistas entered an exciting new phase of her life. I increasingly endorsed the role of grandmother, blessed in short order with four beautiful little grandchildren. I began to write in earnest: some personalized children's books and poems for Kidstories, some freelance articles for several early childhood publications, a memory piece for the New York Times. Life was fulfilling.

I wrote several feature articles for my Internet service provider to post online. When he officially initiated his LI Web-zine, L.I. EYE, I suddenly was thrown full force into the writer's world, as his new co-editor. What wonderful new challenges at this stage of my life!

It was all such fun. I felt excited, stimulated, productive. Ken and I took several nice vacations, attended theater and concerts, enjoyed the camaraderie of our close circle of friends. I felt vital. With an active family life, satisfying social life and new outlets for my creative energies, I was hardly a person propelled toward cosmetic surgery. It never even entered my mind. I still thought of cosmetic surgery as an indulgence reserved for high profile, affluent public personalities. I don't know what my friends thought. We never discussed it. I know for sure none of them had undergone any such procedures.

Time marched on. In retrospect I realize that subliminally some of those creeping signs of age were working on me. I just didn't allow myself to acknowledge them. My newly preferred daily attire included a variety of warm up suits over cotton turtle or mock turtleneck shirts. Increasingly my beautiful open neck silk and faux silk blouses hung in my closet, unworn from season to season. *More comfortable, this way*, I rationalized. *No need to dress up for work any longer. I can just be casually myself.*

Those were the explanations I gave myself. I rarely ventured into the stores to shop for clothes any more. I no longer enjoyed that ritual. I didn't like how I looked in anything. Was it the clothes or the reflection peering back at me from the dressing room mirror?

I was using more concealer under my eyes, but there were days when I would still get a startling jolt when I looked at my reflection. That person staring back at me looked remarkable like my mother. I didn't feel the age of that person. I'd make excuses – tell myself that I just looked tired that day, tell myself that I was pushing too hard, that I really needed to get more sleep.

Ken reinforced my thoughts. He wasn't thrilled with my long hours of concentrated work. "This is supposed to be your retirement – the time for you to take it easy and enjoy life. You're spending too much time sitting in front of the computer. It's showing on your face – you just look so intense." That last sentence reverberated in my ears. It was true enough. But was it my long hours before the computer or was it Father Time creeping up on me?

In the past, I had felt confidant in my ability to convey a more positive image with face-to-face contacts and knew this usually gave me a persuasive advantage. This no longer seemed the case. I began to rely more heavily on telephone and e-mail contacts as a means of communication and placated myself with a pat on the back and self-assurances that I had joined the ranks of the technologically savvy.

Call it rationalization, call it denial, call it what your will. . . but underneath it all, I was conscious of subtle, pinprick reminders about my aging appearance.

The Photograph Episode

My web-zine publisher asked me to write a brief bio and send him a photo to post on-line. One morning I spread out a number of photographs from my recent past on the dinette table. An electrician, working in our kitchen that day, paused to take a look over my shoulder.

"H-m-m, you look pretty there", he said as he pointed to a headshot taken on students' picture day, exactly five years earlier. "And how long ago was that picture taken?" he questioned, not unkindly. "Actually, not that long ago", I answered truthfully. "Well, you must have had a different hairdo or something", he continued.

I looked at that photograph again. My hairstyle was pretty much the same. Actually, at that time I didn't think it an overly flattering picture, but my opinion of it grew stronger over time. Five years later I thought I really looked good back then.

The Invisibility Factor

And then there were those sins of omission from perfect strangers. I felt like a veil of invisibility had descended upon me. I'm not talking sexual innuendo here or overt invitation. I am talking simply about those non-verbal expressions of approval, connection, acceptance. All my life I had experienced welcoming glances, instant smiles, ready eye contact and expressions of approval from people I newly encountered. I felt this missing from my daily life and wondered where it had gone. Had retirement changed me? Was I projecting a hurried, impatient image? Perhaps I was to blame.

I made a conscious effort to reach out with an aura of friendliness. I tried extra hard to make eye contact with the young woman at the cosmetic counter of one of the nearby department stores, but still felt her brush me aside when a pretty, twenty-ish year old sat down beside me.

I gave the clerk at the local post office a warm smile, commented about his barking cough and told him I hoped he felt better. He gave me a half-hearted mumble, looked over my head and called out "Next" to the next patron in line.

Why did I need this kind of validation? Habit, perhaps. Customary expectation? Ghosts of insecurities past? I'm not certain of the answer. But I am certain of my feelings. I felt dismissed, insignificant, invisible. Why should that be? My life had veered off in so many new directions. If anything, probably I was a more interesting person than ever before. Shouldn't that make me feel more attractive? But it didn't. I felt like the dichotomy between my self-perception of the inner me and the outside world's view of me had widened considerably.

Still the thought of cosmetic surgery was far from my consciousness. Most likely I never would have pursued it, had fate not intervened.

Medical Intervention

As a result of a very mild case of shingles, I was left with a condition known as Herpes Zoster, which scarred the cornea of my right eye. As the muscles in that eye continued to weaken, my upper eyelids slackened - first the right lid, then the left, as if to match it. I was finding it increasingly difficult to read.

When I complained to my ophthalmologist, he explained that my condition had caused weakened eye muscles or Ptosis, assured me it could be repaired quite easily with a few stitches to my upper lids and referred me to an ophthalmic surgeon.

I had become so involved with eye treatments - regularly scheduled visits to the corneal specialist, emergency visits as flair ups occurred . . . , that I hadn't focused on the cosmetic aspect. Now I did. Ptosis seemed to have robbed my eyes of their brightness and sparkle. Even their blue color seemed to have faded to a greenish gray. My once prettiest feature now looked unremarkable – tired and dull.

I scheduled an appointment with the ophthalmic surgeon. I didn't know it then, but he would be my first toe step into the world of cosmetic surgery.

What Propels Us

In retrospect I recognized that there were many forces inching me toward cosmetic surgery, but I wasn't open to that thought. It took a catalyst to nudge me forward. That medically necessary surgical repair to my eyelids was the event that started me thinking: "As long as I need to go under anesthesia, why not some cosmetic enhancement at the same time?"

When I asked **Denise** to tell me about her clients' motivations for cosmetic surgery, she talked in terms of two basic motivations for women, the first of which was a desire to enhance their self-image and attractiveness to men.

She explained that many women tell her they decided on cosmetic surgery because they "just can't stand looking in the mirror anymore", but an equal number make that decision because they feel like they have become invisible to men. They talk about the sadness they experience when men look at them to see what was there and then just look away.

"We all have those human needs for love and recognition", said **Denise**, "but I also believe that there is a significant undercurrent of sexuality motivating many women, although they don't always recognize it as such."

What is clear to Denise is that none of the women who come to her are ready to give up on life and use cosmetic surgery as a means to give themselves a second chance.

Carol, the retired math teacher and sports enthusiast you met in Chapter 3, *What Can You Expect After Cosmetic Surgery?,* started to think about having a facelift when she looked down into a mirror and saw an old lady looking back at her. "I wasn't ready to be an old lady. I felt I had too much to do yet and wanted to look as young and energetic as I felt", said **Carol,** whose own mother advised her that she needed a facelift after seeing the results of her dental assistant's cosmetic surgery.

Anne, the registered nurse from Harrisburg, Pa. was suddenly struck by the thought of a facelift while getting dressed to attend the wedding of a family friend. "I put on a beautiful dress, but I somehow just felt frumpy. I noticed my jowls and said to myself: *Anne, you are aging.*" Like other aging women I spoke with, **Anne** found herself overwhelmed by a yearning to regain her youth.

It is often difficult for women to reconcile their aging appearance with the youthful energy they feel. "As I aged, my facial expression just seemed to change", said **Whitney**, a delightful woman from a suburb of Cincinnati, Ohio who just happens to be my granddaughter, Emily's other grandmother. "What I saw in the mirror was an angry expression - very different from the way I felt inside." **Diane**, the warm, caring woman from Chapter 3, *What Can You Expect After Cosmetic Surgery,* who described herself as being "generous in her friendships", also spoke about hating that mirror reflection staring back at her. "I saw slits where my eyes used to be. I had no lids and fatty deposits under my eyes."

When I asked **Denise** if any of her clients spoke about sudden catalysts to their decisions to go for cosmetic surgery, she explained that sometimes a simple event or comment triggers this thought. As an example, she spoke about a fifty-seven year old client named **Janet**, who hired the same painter she had used a decade earlier to come repaint her apartment. As the men worked, she overheard the painter's assistant say: "Isn't she pretty?" and the painter/contractor respond: "Oh, that's nothing, you should have seen her ten years ago." **Janet** called Denise the following week to schedule an appointment.

Denise described a similar event as the catalyst for her client, **Elizabeth**, the young widow who fell in love with a pilot several years after her facelift. When she was forty-six years old, **Elizabeth** and her husband adopted a baby daughter and five years later, entered her in preschool. She overheard a group of the other mothers refer to her as the grandmother, and described that episode as an awakening because it made her realize just how old and haggard she looked.

Carol's catalyst came in the form of a gift after attending a wedding with a group of colleagues. "Later, one of them gave me a 5" X 7" photo of myself taken that evening. I took one look at that picture and thought: *This is a friend? Why would she give me such a terrible photo?"* **Carol** described that picture as a big factor in pushing her forward.

Similarly, a comment from **Whitney's** husband served as a catalyst for her. She explained how she saw a concerned look come across his face as they approached one another from opposite ends of a store. He asked her why she was so angry when actually, to the contrary, she was feeling quite happy. "Well, you looked anything but happy as you were walking toward me", he said. When she got home and looked in the mirror, she saw an angry face, that in no way reflected her inner feelings, staring back at her. Her husband's comment was the catalyst that started **Whitney** on the path to reversing some of those signs of aging..

Some women spoke about that undercurrent of sexuality which **Denise** referred to earlier. **Jane**, a fifty-six year old school administrator and golf enthusiast, explained that when she was in her 20's and 30's men would look at her, try to make conversation with her. "After awhile, I realized that that didn't happen anymore. I kind of felt like I faded into the woodwork."

These thoughts were echoed by **Diane**: "When I was younger, men used to look at me, make eye contact with me. That just wasn't happening anymore. So I guess on one level I wanted that."

Other women spoke of a palpable connection between sexuality and cosmetic surgery. **Donna**, a sixty year old dental assistant for a pediatric dentist, spoke about experiencing a sexual mid-life crisis:

> "I was astounded by the things I discovered about myself which helped me grow and explore in ways I never had done before. I really think there was a connection between my personal sexual awakening

and my desire for cosmetic surgery. I had begun to feel more sexual and I suddenly wanted to be that younger, more sexual woman."

But it was **Tina**, a forty year old woman from Kansas, who nearly made me drop the receiver when she shared her story.

"I usually take top position during sex because my husband is much taller and heavier than me. One night I looked down at my sagging breasts during sex and it just destroyed the mood for me. I wondered how my husband possibly could be enjoying this if I was so turned off by the sight of my body."

It didn't take **Tina** long to make her decision. "That next day, when I thought about how nice it would be to have sex with a new, improved body, I decided to have a breast lift."

I asked **Denise** if many women get encouragement from a spouse, parent or other meaningful person in their lives. Although she said she rarely hears that, she believes that the healthiest motivations for cosmetic surgery are those that come from within. Her advice is: "Each woman should make this decision for herself. She should not choose cosmetic surgery simply to please someone else."

Lauren, the fifty year old woman from Atlanta, Georgia made that decision for herself with no prompting from loved ones.

"My mother, who is in her eighties, still looks unbelievably young except for her very sagging neck. I knew that would be my future so I decided to take things into my own hands and turn back the clock."

In studies by Lerner and Javonovic, we learn that there is often a physical reality to this desire to change an aspect of one's appearance. It is interesting to note that within each subculture, standardized concepts of beauty exist to a surprisingly universal degree. The more a particular feature deviates from its universal standard of beauty, such as the strongly elongated nose or deeply receded chin, the more that person tends to feel conspicuously different or unattractive. **1**

Such was the case for the clinical psychologist, **Rose**, whose nose did not fit with a standardized concept of beauty. Despite her father's conviction that it was an aristocratic nose that should not be changed, she remained unconvinced. "I was always self-conscious about my nose. I wouldn't wear my hair pulled back. When someone met me, I was sure that was the first thing they focused on." But after her nose was broken and healed slightly crooked, **Rose** said she became more determined than ever to get it fixed.

Norma Jean, on the other hand, initially seemed to enjoy the attention her distinctive nose generated. "My nose was a bit Semitic (or Indian or Hispanic) looking and people had a difficult time figuring out where I came from." But she too chose to have a rhinoplasty after her nose began to veer too far from those universal standards of beauty.

> "When I hit forty-five, I noticed my nose had grown and would continue to grow, as my mother's nose had grown. It was then that I decided to have my nose done, but insisted that it be as close to my own as possible."

In addition to facial features, diminished self-esteem often occurs when part of a women's body veers far from universal standards of beauty. Women with breasts of an atypical size or shape are at especially high risk for reduced self-esteem.

Nicole talked about how as a teenager she bought everything she could get her hands on including padded bras, inserts, and duct tape, to give herself some semblance of cleavage. She spoke of the very motherly, feminine feeling she experienced when, after giving birth to her first child, her breasts filled up with milk. She loved the way they looked. But when she stopped nursing, her breasts looked worse than prior to pregnancy.

> "I became so self-conscious that even intimacy with my husband was becoming a problem. I felt embarrassed and hesitant about having my husband see me naked."

On a scale of 1-5, **Nicole** rated her self-consciousness level as minus 2 and began researching breast augmentation surgery during her second pregnancy.

A woman you already met in Chapter 1, *Cosmetic Surgery, The Aphrodisiac Effect,* who had responded to my cosmetic surgery questionnaire with the creative pen name, **Chesty**, wrote about the poor self-esteem she suffered because of her underdeveloped breasts.

> "While I was a teenager, I watched all my friends develop breasts while I remained completely flat. I got lots of teasing in the girl's locker room. One day a girl I never liked, shouted out to me from across the room: 'Hey, ___, how did you get those two little mosquito bites this time of year?'

> "Some of the other girls started to laugh. I just wanted to cry, I felt so embarrassed and inadequate. I never forgot that moment of anguish. I never was able to shed that feeling of self-consciousness about my breasts."

I thought about **Chesty**'s experience when I read a chapter on *Physical Appearance and Society* written by Sarwer and Magee, where they spoke about peer related teasing as one factor furthering popularity of breast enhancing brassieres and augmentation surgeries. 2

As we learned in Chapter 1, *Cosmetic Surgery, The Aphrodisiac Effect,* **Chesty's** underdeveloped breasts were a strong inhibitor when it came to dating and intimate relationships. She ended her story with the words: "Breast augmentation gave me that gift that no amount of therapy ever could have provided."

Unlike **Nicole** and **Chesty**, **MaryLou's** self-esteem suffered from the reverse problem. By the time she was in her late teens, she described her breasts as so pendulous that they almost reached down to her waist.

"From the time I was a teenager, I felt totally embarrassed by my body. I walked with my shoulders slumped forward so people wouldn't notice my breasts and wore oversize blouses and cardigan sweaters to hide what was underneath. During my marriage, I felt so ashamed of my body that it had a bad impact on our relationship."

But it wasn't until about a year after her divorce, that **MaryLou** decided to take charge of her life and had breast reduction surgery. The following year she had liposuction to get rid of her saddlebag thighs. How wonderful to read her last comment: "Now I feel proud of my body instead of embarrassment and shame."

As **Denise** and I continued our discussion about women's motivations for cosmetic surgery, she turned the conversation to another set of motivators – those that involve improvements to one's career or social status. **Denise** explained that women now realize that they can be in control of their destinies.

> "The technology is all out there, just waiting for them. Women are aware that much of the world, both socially and in the work force, is taking advantage of what is available and they don't want to be left behind. In order to face the competition, it just seems like the right thing to do."

I immediately thought of her client, **Pamela**, the photographer you met in Chapter 4, *Preferential Treatment For the Pretty Ones,* whose career blossomed along with her appearance after cosmetic surgery.

Internal and External Motivators

Internal and external motivations for cosmetic surgery have been discussed for decades. An example of an internal motivator would be a desire to increase self-confidence and self-esteem through an improved physical appearance, such as was apparent in the words expressed by **Chesty**, **Rose**, **MaryLou**, **Nicole**, **Diane** and **Jane**. An example of an external motivator would be a desire to improve one's career or social status in life.

Sydney, a sixty year old woman who had a full facelift to keep her competitive edge as a realtor, is a perfect example of the external type motivator described above.

> "When I noticed that I wasn't commanding as many clients as the younger women in my office, I attributed it to my aging appearance. I decided to have cosmetic surgery to remain competitive in my profession."

Interestingly, **Sydney** got more than she had hoped for.

> "My client list did grow after my surgery, but my spirits also surged. I feel like I came back to life. People notice me again and smile at me. I radiate renewed energy in my work and in my personal life."

Kristen also underwent a facelift to reverse the pattern of a waning career in computer technology, an area she described as a very male dominated field at that time. When she was in her late twenties and early thirties, she had full attendance at her training sessions, but by age forty-eight she noticed this was no longer the case.

Concern for her career motivated her to have a facelift, a reason that would fit right into the category of an external motivator; but when you listen to the rest of **Kristen's** story, you will realize that part of her motivation was internal with sexual overtones:

> "A big part of my job entailed travel to train others in the application of the newest applications of work related software. When I was in my late 20's and early 30's, I would watch men enter a training session with a disgruntled expression, take a look at me or my partner and suddenly liven up. It was like they had made a snap judgment about us, that we would be good presenters, just because we were attractive women. Afterwards, men would come up to us to praise our presentation, but sometimes I felt like it was just an excuse to engage in private conversation.'

> "We got lots of compliments then. Oh, yes, we got offers too, but we were very careful about that. Shortly after my forty-seventh birthday, before one of my workshops, I heard one of the men whisper to his buddy, 'Let's go down the hall. There's a real looker presenting in Conference Room C.'
> That hurt. It was like being told that my value as a professional faded along with my looks. At the end of that day, my partner turned to me and said: 'Do you notice something? Nobody is making offers anymore.' We laughed, but it was a bittersweet moment at the end of a bittersweet day."

Again, in their segment on *Physical Appearance and Society*, Sarwer and Magee note that:

"Women are rated less feminine as they grow older whereas men's ratings of masculinity do not vary with age." **3**

As women continue to age, many find it difficult to reconcile their inner feelings of femininity with decreased attention they tend to receive in the outside world. Interestingly, many people, including **Sydney** and **Kristen**, think they are having cosmetic surgery for pragmatic reason, but discover other motivations under the surface and occasional unexpected benefits along the way.

Gail shared an article about a fifty-eight year old business woman who originally listed pragmatics as her motivation for cosmetic surgery, but later reconsidered and gave this more studied response.

> "I didn't tell you the most important thing. When you get to be my age, people stop noticing you. That's everybody, anywhere. You become a non-person. After my facelift, people noticed me again. They noticed me being alive. I became a person again." **4**

The above quote is one woman's testimony to both motivators at work: the external motivator, to remain competitive in the work world and the internal motivator, to be noticed once again. As we have seen, this latter thought is one often voiced by women middle age and beyond.

As further examples of externally motivated women, I share the stories from two who used cosmetic surgery as a vehicle to please their husbands. **Janine** was quite upfront in her admission that financial security is important to her, but that as an airline employee, her income is limited.

"I don't want to live the lifestyle I could afford on my income, but my husband is a very good provide. As long as I'm married to him, my salary isn't a necessity. Since my first cosmetic surgery, my husband has kept after me to have more and more. I don't even want most of it, but I do it to keep him happy. He's really insecure and having a pretty wife inflates his ego. If this is what it takes to make our marriage work, I'm willing to go along with it."

Fifty-four year old **Lucy** also had cosmetic surgery to please her husband. "I am ten years older than my husband. Let's face it, he could get a younger woman if he wanted to. I had a facelift because I didn't want to lose him." Both **Janine** and **Lucy** were externally motivated. Although they already reached one of their life goals, they used cosmetic surgery as a means to try to maintain the positions they had achieved.

Denise agreed that sometimes motivations are more complex. She referred to **Alisa**, a Colorado native who was locked into an unhealthy martial relationship. **Alisa** used cosmetic surgery as a vehicle both to regain her self-respect and to generate enough courage to leave an abusive husband in order to begin life anew.

As a final category **Denise** spoke about clients who have used cosmetic surgery as a reward after either undergoing a difficult life experience or reaching a specific milestone, as a special birthday or after achieving long sought weight goals.

Hewitt is one such example. One evening, after reading about my study in our college alumni magazine, she called me from Florida, proudly introducing herself as a ten year survivor of ovarian cancer. Here is her story:

> "After surgery for my ovarian cancer, I said I needed a big treat for myself and getting rid of a turkey neck and huge double chin was going to be it. I waited for one year after treatment was done and began interviewing surgeons. I thought if I could go through cancer treatment, this cosmetic surgery would not be too bad. I was surprised that my MD did not think this was an odd treat for surviving cancer."

Secret Motivations

It will probably not surprise you to learn that some women have motivations for surgery that they don't fully understand or motivations they understand, but do not disclose to their surgeons. In a study of fifty female facelift patients, the researchers discovered that over half of the patients revealed unrealistic or secret motivations to the researcher, which they concealed from their surgeons. 5

One group of women gave their surgeons details of their aging appearance as the motivation for surgery, but when speaking privately to the researcher or when helped to explore their deeper motivations, expressed an underlying fear of aging, which represented not merely deterioration of physical appearance, but abandonment of friends, family and society in general. For these women, cosmetic surgery was a means to retain relationships of love, visibility and involvement.

Another group, sought cosmetic surgery as a means to fix problems in their marital relationships such as to reawaken a husband's interest – even to cure one husband's erectile dysfunction, which of course never materialized – when a prescription of Viagra or Cialis might have been a simpler, more effective solution!

In a different study, out of forty-two patients who listed 'preparation for a life change' as their motivation for surgery, four of them obtained a legal separation or divorce within six months after their surgeries. 6

Diane spoke of one friend whose marriage wasn't going so well.

> "When she had a facelift, I asked her if she did this to make her husband more interested, more physically attracted to her. Her first response was

'no', but then she reconsidered and said, 'Well, maybe'."

Anne concurred by sharing her surgeon's observations about post cosmetic surgery impacts on some marriages:

> "My surgeon told me that after cosmetic surgery, some of his female patients leave their husbands for younger men. That's not me, but I thought it was an interesting comment."

An undercurrent of sexuality, a desire to be noticed and admired by men, is implicit in the content of many of the interviews I conducted. Although **Tina** recognized sexuality up front as her primary motivation, other women including **Donna** and **Anne** began to consciously recognize the relationship between sexuality and their desire for cosmetic surgery as we spoke together. Perhaps it is more of a motivating force than any of us recognize.

In his book, *Listening to Prozak*, Peter Kramer, MD, notes that some people use cosmetic surgery psychiatrically. **7** Although none of my women respondents came anywhere near using cosmetic surgery as a substitute for Prozak, it is clear that with increased self-esteem, some discovered improvement in interpersonal and intimate relationships, dating, careers and other endeavors. But, as you will see when you read Chapter 9, *Secrecy, Deception and Lies*, those whose expectations remain unrealized after cosmetic surgery can experience severe disappointment.

> "Body image is central to plastic surgery as nearly every chapter in this volume articulates. Most cosmetic surgery patients are seeking improvement to their body image but not necessarily on other aspects of psychosocial quality of life. They want to feel more positively about specific aspects of their appearance. For others, the changes they desire may

be more pervasive, as to alter one's self-concept. A small minority of people look to cosmetic surgery for life transformation – more often than not a misguided and ineffective solution." **8**

Helpful Resources

See also the following end-of-book helpful resources pertinent to information found in this chapter.

CD Part C: Self-Assessment Quiz - Are You a Good Candidate for Cosmetic Surgery

CD Part I: Test Your Body Image

Appendix 8: Personal Profiles
(More about the people whose names appear in this chapter)

Appendix 9: Additional Stories for Chapter 7

Footnotes

1. Lerner RM. and Javonovic J. "The role of body image in psychosocial development across the lifespan: A developmental contextual perspective". In Cash TF. and Pruzinsky (Eds.). Body Image: Development, Deviance and Change. New York: Guilford (1990).

2. Sarwer DB. La Rossa D. and Bartlett SP. et al. "Body image concerns of breast augmentation patients". Plastic Reconstructive Surgery. In. Psychological Aspects of Reconstructive and Cosmetic Plastic. Plastic Reconstructive Surgery. 112 (2003): 83-90.

3. Deutsch FM Zalenski CM and Clark ME. "Is there a double standard of aging?" Journal of Applied Social Psychology. 16 (1986): 771-785.

4. Hamburger A and Hall H. "Beauty Quest." Psychology Today. 22.5 (1988): 28(5).

5. Goin MK. Burgoyne RW. Goin JM. and Staples FR. "A prospective psychological study of 50 female face-lift patients". Plastic and Reconstructive Surgery (1980): 436-442.

6. Belfer ML. "Cosmetic surgery as an antecedent of life change." American Journal of Psychiatry. 136. 199-201.

7. Kramer P. Listening to Prozak: The Landmark Book About Antidepressants and the Remaking of the Self. Penguin Books. (1994). DIANE Publishing Company. (1998).

8. Cash TF. "Psychology of physical appearance". In. Sarwer DB. et al. eds. Psychological Aspects of Reconstructive and Cosmetic Plastic Surgery: Clinical, Empirical and Ethical Perspectives. Lippincott, Williams and Wilkens. (2005): 37.

The Short Story:
Women's roadblocks and obstacles to cosmetic surgery

"Roadblocks: Thoughts or events that deter action"

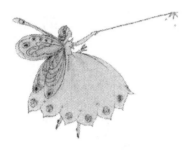

That medically necessary surgical repair to my eyelids became my rationalization for doing more. After all, didn't it make sense, while under anesthesia, to have some cosmetic work done at the same time?

On the drive home, after the last of three consultations, I kept thinking: *Me? Is this really me?* To help rid myself of my ambivalences, I began to invent some imaginary conversations. The first one was with my mom, about what she would say now, if only able to speak with her former eloquence:

> *Lois, why are you even entertaining such thoughts? Is it so important to you that you're even willing to have surgery just to get rid of a few wrinkles? I think you look lovely, just the way you are. You know, I've always had such respect for your judgment. You're*

such an intelligent person - so level headed – that I'm really surprised you're thinking this way now. This doesn't even sound like something you would do. If you want my advice, forget it. Remember, sometimes when you look for trouble, trouble finds you.

I laughed aloud as I continued with an invented, yet true-to-form conversation with my dad:

How much is this going to cost you? What a crazy idea! You could take that money and add to a college fund for your grandchildren, invest in a good quality mutual fund. Then your money could work for you. You could do something sensible, something to help your family, instead of spending money to have your face cut apart. For God sake, people do everything they can to avoid surgery and you're going to do this for no good reason. Isn't Kenny happy with you the way you are? What are you trying to do, look for a new boyfriend at this stage in your life?

I put their voices aside to listen to my own. *Lois, trust your instincts*, it whispered in my ear. I clearly needed to work through some ambivalent feelings before I could make a comfortable decision for myself.

Although I approached my mental roadblocks in a rather whimsical way, my invented conversation actually helped me work through some of the obstacles I had set for myself through my parents lingering voices:

- Cosmetic surgery is an act of vanity.
- Don't subject yourself to unnecessary surgery.
- Use your intelligence to better advantage.
- Learn to grow old gracefully.
- Don't look for trouble.
- Spend your money sensibly - not frivolously or selfishly.
- Sexuality shouldn't be an issue at your age.

As I interviewed other women, I repeatedly heard variations of those refrains. Some expressed concern about what others would think. **Carol** even worried that people might suspect that she was having a facelift so soon after her husband's death in order to replace him, when actually her surgery had been planned with his full approval the year before his untimely death.

In her questionnaire response, **Carmella** wrote about feeling that she was doing something shameful.

> "It's a shame women feel plastic surgery is a 'back door' issue. When I went for my consultation, many women in the surgeon's waiting room kept to themselves and looked down. I wanted to leave because it made me feel as if I was doing something 'bad'."

When I asked **Denise** if her clients express many fears or concerns prior to surgery, she explained that the greatest concern they express is fear that they will be unhappy with the results. To reassure them, she often puts them in touch with other clients who have undergone similar procedures with the same surgeon. Occasionally she hears women talk about feeling guilty they are spending so much money on themselves. **Denise** advises these women to think of cosmetic surgery as an investment in themselves and reminds them of her favorite slogan: *Youth and Beauty are Power Tools.*

Women Who Don't Want Cosmetic Surgery

I wondered what thoughts, fears and belief systems deterred other woman from having cosmetic surgery. I decided to interview several of them who had voiced their own resistance to it. Four of these women are personal friends, one, referred through a friend. I had specific criteria in mind. I wanted to speak with women who were intelligent, attractive, financially stable and age fifty-five or above, so that those inevitable signs of aging would have at least begun to emerge. I purposely avoided selecting young women with out-of- norm features, for fear that such choices would be interpreted as negative statements about their appearance.

The first two women you will meet initially spoke about the financial aspect, the costs involved in cosmetic surgery. First on my list was **Jenny Jasper**.

We became friends in college and have maintained a close friendship for over forty years. She was born into a family of well-respected political activists, who have dedicated much of their lives to improving benefits and rights for the less fortunate. **Jenny** currently is employed as Director of Health Care Services for Women and is an ardent supporter of a woman's right to choose. She is well informed on practically any topic that flows from our spirited conversations, thoughtful yet quick witted. Her home is piled high with books, magazines and newspapers, which she manages to find time to devour despite her busy schedule.

A most attractive woman with auburn hair, finely chiseled features and a once porcelain like complexion, time and years of smoking have brought wrinkles to this still pretty face.

Jenny expressed a temptation to do something to erase some of those signs of aging on her face. When I asked what deterred her, she told me that if she had unlimited funds, she'd probably consider it, "but there are so many other things I would rather do than a fixed up face". For example, she thought travel was much more important to her.

Next I want you to meet **Harriet Spitzer**, a more recent friend, whom I met shortly after I had accepted a position as chairperson of the NYSUT (New York State Reading Association) Pre-conference Institute for their annual conference. I was so taken by her enthusiasm, intellect and expertise that I invited her to participate as one of our presenters.

Harriet has worked as both an educator and a college administrator. She also has an ardent interest in politics, captured perfectly in a press photo of her as a young mother nursing her infant son while simultaneously serving as delegate to the 1972 Democratic National Convention.

Harriet's long dark hair is simply but attractively styled, colored to compliment her complexion. She keeps her trim body in shape through regular workouts at the gym. I would describe her attire as fashionable, yet tailored.

When I asked **Harriet** why she would not consider cosmetic surgery for herself, like **Jenny**, she first spoke about the financial aspect.

> "Well, first of all, it's a lot of money - I imagine at least $15,000 for a facelift. I ask myself, if I do that, spend that kind of money, what do I give up? I can think of a lot of other things more meaningful to my life."

Few of us have unlimited funds. I chose a facelift instead of a trip to China. Both **Jenny** and **Harriet** were telling me they had set other priorities.

As I continued my conversations with each of them, other issues continued to emerge. **Jenny** talked about her background, that her parents always stressed the importance of one's mission in life, that they taught her through their living example that we are here on Earth to do good for others.

> "So cosmetic surgery just doesn't fit with the thinking side of me. I imagine I would think of

myself as slightly frivolous even though I know it's okay to be frivolous."

Harriet also expressed thoughts about her value system. She spoke of her awareness of our superficial society with its emphasis on beauty, but that for her, achievement was far more significant.

> "If you were born beautiful or have had something done to make yourself look more beautiful, you haven't had to do much to achieve that. But if you choose to become more educated, more accomplished, that takes effort. Then you can give back to others. If you have enriched yourself, then you can enrich others. That to me is the real measure of a person. On my value scale, that's terrific. The other stuff is further down on the scale."

Jenny, on the other hand, talked about aesthetics, that she likes to look at beautiful things, loves clothes, would love to look better. "I guess it all comes down to finances and the psychology of it all – to justify spending that kind of money on myself."

As you will discover when you read my Epilogue, I spoke nearly those identical words when I whispered to a friend: "I think I'd really like to do this for myself, but I'm finding it hard to justify such an ego-centric expense."

My route to cosmetic surgery was circuitous at best, as a medically necessary repair to my eyelids is what started the whole process in motion for me. **Jenny** instinctively understood:

> "If I were like you and had a rationalization, a medical reason, to fix something, then I'd go ahead and have a facelift at the same time, and would have no problem with my mother."

Hold on to **Jenny's** last comment about her mother. We will return to it and to other thoughts from both **Jenny** and **Harriet** after you meet my next two interview subjects.

I spent two hours on the phone with my friend **Rita Spina**, exploring some of her thoughts. **Rita**, a past chairperson of the psychology department in the school district where I once worked, is one of the most universally adored people I know. A skilled psychologist with a caring heart, sense of adventure, innovative spirit, fun loving nature; she is also a published author and noted artist who frequently exhibits at juried shows. She is tall, slender and physically attractive. When I first met **Rita**, she was spectacularly beautiful.

During our conversation, there was no mention of finances, but **Rita's** fear of anesthesia loomed large. She told me a harrowing story about her sister, Suzanne, who as a young girl, needed surgery to repair an infected tear duct. She was given sodium pentathol in the physician's office.

> "It was a new anesthesia at the time. Suzanne went into anaphylactic shock and never recovered. I know they have improved on various forms of anesthesia today, but that fear has stayed with me."

I asked **Rita** if she would consider cosmetic surgery if it could be done without anesthesia. "Sure, but it can't", she answered. She told me that some years ago, she had considered having her eyes done and had several consultations with plastic surgeons.

> "My eyes were always my most outstanding feature, the thing that others noticed and commented about when I was younger, but I never went through with the surgery."

She then spoke more about how her fear of anesthesia resurfaced when she needed some major dental work:

"It took me awhile, but I finally let my periodontist do the work under a mild anesthesia. I knew that otherwise I would lose all my teeth. I guess I need a strong enough incentive to overcome my anxiety, and saving my teeth was quite a motivator."

I commented on the fact that she always had dynamite eyes, then digressed as I recalled a story she had shared with me years earlier.

> "I remember you telling me a story about a day when Larry was fixing your hair and suddenly you had this fantasy image of yourself – that you would look in the mirror after he was finished and see this ravishing beauty staring back at you. You and Larry had a good laugh over that at the time."

I told **Rita** I thought she was still a very attractive woman, but wondered if she ever thought about recapturing the youthful glow of that ravishing beauty she envisioned in the mirror that day.

Rita expressed her personal feelings of ambivalence.

> "Well, I don't like it, but I say to myself: *You're just going to be you.* I'm sometimes in conflict about this. Why do I have to change who I am? I resist that."

She spoke about how long it took before she wore contacts and yet that she is very conscious of how she dresses, wears flattering colors and likes to put herself together well. If she gains a couple of pounds, she immediately steps back and takes them off. "I've always been told how attractive I am, so I have that going for me. I tell myself, *I am good enough.*"

Jenny expressed similar feelings of ambivalence. She told me that she didn't think cosmetic surgery would make a huge difference in her life. "People who love me will still love me. I would be the one to feel better", she said. But she also recognized the importance of feeling better about oneself. "I'm the first to say that it is a very important thing, feeling good about yourself."

We will return to **Rita**, **Jenny** and **Harriet** in a short while. But first I want you to get reacquainted with **Dorothy Birnham**, a woman you first met in Chapter 1, *Cosmetic Surgery - The Aphrodisiac Effect*, where she shared her thoughts about physical appearance and marital opportunities.

Dorothy lives in a suburb of Chapel Hill, North Carolina - and, to date, we have only met through phone conversations. It was **Rita** who spoke to Dorothy about my project and matched us up as a good fit. I found her to be not only a delightful conversationalist and an outgoing, friendly person; but also perceptive, interesting and conscientious about her contributions to our discussions. We had two lengthy phone interview sessions. By now we feel more friends than voices transmitted across the wires.

Although **Dorothy** shared her fears of both anesthesia and surgery, her concerns seemed less focused on the life threatening aspects expressed by **Rita** than on two different concerns. For one thing, she knew she would suffer tremendous anxiety in the days before the surgery: "I'm a real coward when I go for any kind of office visits. I have 'white coat syndrome'. My blood pressure actually goes up, I get that nervous."

Jenny had spoken about her *fear of the knife* and her superstition that *we shouldn't tempt the fates*. **Dorothy** spoke similarly. She explained that when she was young, doctors in her family repeatedly talked about "not going under the knife, under anesthesia, unless it's an absolute necessity" and she said that that thought still impacts on her.

"If I could press a button and have it done, sure, I'd do it", she said. But of course there is no such button. **Rita** would have had an eyelift if the procedure could have been done without anesthesia. But that too is not currently feasible. Secondly, **Dorothy** spoke of the same concern that **Denise** mentioned earlier as the one she most often hears voiced by her clients - concern about the surgical results.

Dorothy talked about her friend **Ricki**, who went to Florida to have cosmetic surgery with a surgeon who is supposed to have a great reputation. Although the surgery went well, her friend's neck never healed quite right. She returned to her surgeon three times and each time he tried to fix it, but finally said he couldn't do any more. It was just the nature of her skin, nothing that the surgeon did wrong.

> "Don't get me wrong, she looks gorgeous, but she never dresses without a scarf around her neck. There's always that little concern that things won't go quite right."

Toward the end of our interview, **Dorothy** critiqued society's emphasis on appearance versus recognition and appreciation for the more dynamic aspects of one's personality and character:

> "There's a real dichotomy here. I said looking good fans one's ego so that's one part of it. But there should be more value to a person than just appearance. I love to do hundreds of things. I have a good sense of humor. I'm enthusiastic, full of energy and have good health. My friends are similar. They are just a terrific group of women. If a man meets me or one of my terrific friends, I would want him to feel fortunate to know such a vibrant person. Otherwise I'd think he's just foolish to be unable to recognize the inner value of that person. That's the other side to ego."

Now we know that **Dorothy**, **Jenny** and **Rita** all have ambivalent feelings about cosmetic surgery. I understand completely. I did too.

In her closing statement, Dorothy spoke about her mother:

> "My mom was an egomaniac about how she looked. She was very beautiful and appearance was the most important thing in her life. While I was proud to have a mother who looked the way she did, my emphasis in life was quite different than hers."

Do you remember when **Jenny** said that if there was a medically necessary component for her, she would have cosmetic surgery and then she would have no problem with her mother? I find it interesting to note that **Rita** also ended her interview with a spontaneous reference to her mother:

> "I'm not a particularly vain person. My mother was always focused on the external. I never wanted to be like my mother. I made that separation long ago."

There is no getting around it - in positive and negative ways, as women we are deeply impacted by the patterns our mothers established before us.

Last of all I would like you to meet **Linda Novick**, a retired guidance counselor from the same school district where I once worked. Because I was responsible for the administration of student educational evaluations, including the students assigned to her, we had frequent opportunities to conference together. I looked forward to our joint sessions, where she routinely brought her intelligence, rational judgment and calm, gentle manner to the table.

Tall and physically attractive, **Linda** has a beautiful smile and exudes a quiet confidence. She keeps her graying hair neatly cut and closely cropped, with what I suspect is more a concern for convenience than high style. She had told me that although she was not judgmental about people who underwent cosmetic surgery, she would never take this step for herself. During our interview session, **Linda** expressed absolutely no conflicted feelings.

Her personal belief that we should be defined by our inner beauty and accomplishments, rather than surface appearances, is rock solid.

> "We all do things to satisfy our vanity. We all want to look good. We diet even if we are not obese, dress nicely, exercise. I know exercising has an impact on health, but it also impacts on appearance, how our body looks."

Harriet seemed to agree.

"It's nice to be attractive, but that's too extreme. We go to hairdressers, exercise and diet, buy nice clothes; but cosmetic surgery goes way beyond. It's just excessive."

Linda went on to discuss concerns about anesthesia similar to those already expressed by **Rita** and **Dorothy**. "Every time you go under anesthesia, there is a risk." She said she had this same concern when her husband, Larry, had back surgery, because it was somewhat elective. "But he was in such pain that he couldn't even stand up in the shower so it became a quality of life issue that made it a risk worth taking."

Harriet felt similarly. Her husband Mike had fought a battle with head and neck cancer. "If you have to have surgery to save your life, of course, do it, but not to elect to have surgery."

(Note: Be sure to read the results of my research on safety and cosmetics surgery in Chapter 10, *Misperceptions and Misconceptions,* which presents both cautions and reassurances.)

Linda shared **Harriet's** squeamishness over medical/surgical procedures. "I could never be a doctor. I get queasy just thinking about the whole process - cutting my face apart, pulling up the skin. I just can't deal with the thought of it."

Next **Linda** brought up the feminist issue with the question: "Why do women need to look younger and more attractive and not men? I might be wrong, but I think it is mostly women who go for cosmetic surgery." Linda is correct. The latest statistics show that approximately 90% of all cosmetic procedures nationwide are performed on women.

She said that she believes society puts pressure on women to keep up their appearances, noting that most graying women color their hair, but not the men.

> "Why is it acceptable for the men to let their hair turn white and not the women? I know one's self-image plays a part in that decision, but those outside pressures are just as great. Self-image is so influenced by feedback."

I asked **Linda** what she envisions when she thinks of herself and the aging process.

> "I want to age the way nature intended. I've earned all these lines and wrinkles. It's part of my character. I see a different beauty in that aging face. It shows a strength in character. This is me. I don't have to disguise me in any way."

Harriet's next answers were so remarkable similar that one might suspect that they had compared notes, but I know they did not. "I have lines on my face and all those lines are lines I have earned. They belong to me."

She spoke about a visiting professor at NYIT (New York Institute of Technology) who was an eminent scholar of composition and theory.

> "As I got to know her, I saw that she had such comfort in who she was. She had tremendous assurance - a sense of self, bred from her achievements, which were impressive. When her

picture appeared in the school newspaper, it captured her face. I thought she looked beautiful with all those lines and her gray hair. That's who she was - an older, accomplished woman."

I wanted to clarify one common misperception because I know many people think of cosmetic surgery purely an act of vanity. But I have come to understand that this choice goes so much deeper than most people realize. I explained that it has helped so many women become more fully optimized.

> "Some women tell me that they have been able to achieve more, accomplish more, become more productive people and happier too because they feel so much better about themselves after cosmetic surgery."

I asked Harriet, how she would respond to those thoughts?"

> "I'm sure it's true that looking better makes one feel better and that can translate, for some, to enhanced self-confidence and yes, more accomplishment.'

> "If someone is unhappy about the way she looks and cosmetic surgery offers a quick and easy solution to her unhappiness, she ought not to hesitate about the procedure. I'm aware that good looking people have an easier time of it in our culture than do unattractive people. However, people are also attractive because they are interesting, energetic and passionate about the life they have chosen to lead. For me, attractiveness that is bred in ideas and engagement is more powerful and ultimately more seductive."

Linda again reflected **Harriet's** thoughts:

> "Vanity can be a physical thing, but vanity also can be based on other things. Some people get more satisfaction and self-esteem from what they

accomplish in life than in how they look. Isn't it really our inner beauty that defines us and matters much more than our only "skin deep" outer beauty? Perhaps if we concentrated more on our accomplishments than our appearances, this world would be a better place."

Although **Jenny**, **Rita** and **Dorothy** were somewhat attracted to cosmetic surgery in concept, even if not in relation to themselves, it clearly lacked a seductive tug for either **Harriet** or **Linda**.

Think Time

You might find your voice amongst one of the five women you have just met. Perhaps like Harriet and Linda, you know cosmetic surgery is not for you. Or on the other hand, you might be certain that it is a good choice for you. But if you are experiencing feelings of ambivalence, you are not alone. Here is a little exercise you might want to try if you need to sort through and clarify your thoughts:
I call it **Plus - Minus - Interesting.**

Fold a paper in thirds to form three columns. Label your first column with the heading **Plus**, your second column **Minus** and your third column, **Interesting**. Record all your thoughts and arguments in favor of cosmetic surgery in your first column. What benefits do you expect to gain? How do you think it might make you feel? Is this important to you? Why? Do you hope something in your life might change if you had cosmetic surgery? What would that be?

Record all your thoughts and arguments against cosmetic surgery in your second column. What are your concerns? Do you hold any personal beliefs incompatible with the idea of cosmetic surgery? Do you have any fears? How rational are your fears? Do you have any medical or emotional condition that might complicate your surgical outcome? Will the expense of cosmetic surgery have a devastating effect on your financial stability?

Use the **Interesting** column to record any other thoughts that occur to you, which relate to your feelings about cosmetic surgery, but aren't decidedly Plus or Minus. Read over your entire list once and then file it someplace accessible like in your underwear drawer. Don't look at it again for at least 24 hours.

Evaluate

In the next day or two, when you go for fresh underwear, take out your list and read through it again - but not silently, voice each thought aloud. You might even decide to add more items to one of your columns.

If you have ambivalent thoughts, this little exercise can help you enter into a debate with yourself, take opposite points of view, explore your rational and irrational beliefs. You might even discover that voices from the past, especially those carried over from childhood, are interfering with your ability to form an independent decision. Use both your powers of rational and intuitive thinking to discover where your mind and heart lie. **Plus - Minus - Interesting** can help you become the decision maker in this process.

A further tip from my psychologist friend **Lorraine**:

> "Take a good look at your position in life. Make sure your desire for cosmetic change is grounded in reality. If you have other unresolved problems or if you are truly depressed, you should first consider therapy rather than surgery. What will it really take to make you feel like the whole person you want to be? Remember: *To thine own self be true*."

Cosmetic surgery is not for everyone and you certainly shouldn't do it to please someone else. But, on the other hand, you shouldn't feel embarrassed or ashamed if you think it is a good choice for you. Only you can make that decision for yourself. If in doubt, think it through carefully so that ultimately you can make the right choice for you.

Chapter 9: Secrecy, Deception and Lies

The Short Story:

Why so many choose to remain mute

"Secrecy: A means of keeping knowledge from others"
"Deception: A means of misleading, an illusion or fraud"
"Lie: A false statement"

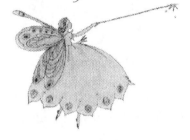

I'm somewhat of a chameleon. Despite the fact that I shared my secret openly with close friends and family, I felt self-conscious about my surgery and considered it a very private matter. Here are a few early events I recall:

About a month after my surgery, my Brazilian neighbor, **Augusta**, dropped in for an evening chat. Seated opposite me in the kitchen, deep in conversation, she suddenly turned dramatically exuberant. "Oh, what hoppen' to you?" she shouted as she jumped up from the table. "What do you mean?" I asked although I had a pretty good idea where she was headed. "You look so beau-tee-ful – your eyes, your skin, your hair", she continued with flamboyant gestures. "Maybe I never sit across from you before. Maybe I never notice."

Ken left the room in a hurry. I laughed but never said anything more. Brazil is a hotbed country for cosmetic surgery, so I knew that if anyone would understand plastic surgery, it would be a Brazilian woman. But I chose to remain mute.

Shortly thereafter, **Harriet Spitzer**, the woman whom I later interviewed at length for Chapter 8, *What Deters Us*, approached me and asked how I was feeling. "Fine", I answered. "Why?" "Oh, just wondering", she responded discretely. I detected her wavelength and surmised who had given her this information.

I called my suspected informer the next day and had my suspicions confirmed. "Have you told anyone else?" I asked. I was horrified to learn that she had. I felt embarrassed, betrayed. "Look", I said. "This is my private business, mine to share or not share as I see fit. I don't want you or Tom to speak of this to anyone. Will you please explain that to him." "Lois, you are absolutely right", she said. "I'm so sorry. I certainly will tell Tom as well."

My book group was another story. **Vivian** and **Harriet W.** already knew. After some time, I told **Alfina**, but cautioned her not to discuss this at our next gathering.

> "Lois, I was looking at you at our last meeting and knew you looked wonderful. It crossed my mind momentarily that maybe you had some work done, but then discounted it. Of course I won't tell anyone, but I wish you could go beyond that. No one is going to think any less of you. Why shouldn't we each have the freedom to do whatever pleases us, as long as we don't hurt anyone in the process. Belly button rings, pierced noses, purple hair . . . , if that's your choice, there's nothing wrong with that. It's *you* who feels uncomfortable about what you did. No one else will judge you harshly, and I think it would help you to talk about it."

At our next meeting, she squeezed my leg during lunch and whispered: "It's okay, tell your story." So I did, while Alfina held my hand under the table. No one seemed the least critical, but then again, they are a special group of women.

And so, little by little I continued to share my story. It was a process I worked through one person at a time. When I wrote my first introduction, I included the words:

> *"Negative vibes often prompt us women to remain mute, to invent all manner of deception to shroud our surgical experiences behind a veil of secrecy. It makes me wonder, when it comes to aesthetics, where do we draw the line between the acceptable, even admirable, and that which evokes cryptic thoughts? Why do we draw that line? Should there be any line at all?"*

Then I sat back on my righteous haunches until I came face to face with an article posted in the Act II section of Newsday. A woman by the name of **Rochelle** had contacted their editor. She wanted to have a facelift, but feared the pain and asked if anyone out there could respond to her concerns. I wanted to reach out to her, to allay her fears, but did I really want my surgery to be a matter of public record?

Then I spoke to myself.

> *Self,* I said, *if you really believe your own words, take that next step and speak up for your beliefs.*

The next day I submitted a letter to Newsday about my experience. I signed it: *Lois W. Stern*

I asked **Denise** if her clients often remain secretive about their surgeries. She explained that some of her clients are high profile people, who don't want the media to track details of their personal lives and therefore arrange to meet her at an undisclosed location to avoid unwarranted publicity. As for her other clients, some go to great lengths to keep the deception alive, whereas others want to tell the world.

None of the women I interviewed seemed to want to tell the world. Most of them opted for varying degrees of secrecy. That beautiful hairstylist, **Val**, spoke about judgmental attitudes she hears around her everyday.

> "I know that for a lot of people, once they hear that someone has had surgery, they say things like: 'Of course she looks good. You'd look good too if you had as much work done on you as she has had on her.' I just hate the thought of people making judgments about me based on cosmetic surgery. That's why I don't tell people about my surgery. If I'm confronted, I admit it, but I hate it - I hate being confronted."

Val thinks it's unfair to judge looking young and attractive by surgery alone because we all know that looking good and feeling good goes way beyond surgery. She named diet, attitude, style and LOTS OF EXERCISE as critical.

Dee, a veterinary assistant from L.I., had a similar story to share. While at a wedding, she sensed 'attitude' from a cousin after she commented favorably about the appearance of another relative. She heard a snicker in her cousin's voice as she said the very words **Val** fears most: "Why shouldn't she look good? She's had a lot of work done on her, if you know what I mean." **Dee** said she wanted to say, 'Good for her. I did too', but when she saw that critical smile come across her cousin's face, she kept silent.

Attitudes toward cosmetic surgery sometimes border on hostility. **Diane**, the delightful woman who goes on a 'girl's vacation' with some of the female members of her family each summer, told the story of a friend who had a facelift while her husband was undergoing treatment for cancer. Her cousin's comment: "With Alex so sick, that's all she has to think about?" implied that this friend was a self-centered, uncaring woman. "She is not that way at all", said **Diane**. "I think she was just trying to lift her spirits during a very difficult time." **Diane** explained that that's why she has been so selective about whom she tells. "I just didn't want that kind of image. I know it shouldn't be like that, but I do care what others think."

As you have noticed, I no longer mind speaking about my cosmetic surgery, but I still don't like the feeling of others talking about me behind my back. **Anne**, the Registered Nurse from Harrisburg, Pa. understood. She told her family and close friends, but downplayed it at work by telling her co-workers that she was having sinus surgery. "I don't share much about my personal life with my co-workers. I just don't like that grapevine effect and hoped it wouldn't be noticed." Fortunately, she didn't have to deal with gossip. Only one person guessed the truth and said: 'I don't know what you had done, but you look fabulous.'

Carmella, the reading specialist with a penchant for ballroom dancing, only told her three closest friends about her tummy tuck and liposuction. Everyone else says, 'Carmella, you keep losing weight', but she just thanks them and says nothing more. "Women can become very catty and sometimes jealous when you look good. I didn't want to deal with that", she explained.

Rose, the clinical psychologist who had her nose fixed, told the people close to her, but didn't make any big announcements. She was getting her doctorate at the time and did a presentation with the bandages still on her nose because she didn't have a choice. If she didn't do it that day, she wouldn't have gotten her degree. She said she didn't feel particularly self-conscious before this women's group, but that it just depends on whom she is talking to.

"Some of my women clients are very conservative and say things like: 'Why would anyone put poison in their bodies?' when they talk about Botox.

Rose feels that people are ignorant about a lot of things, don't bother to get the facts but just make off handed comments to fit in with what they think is the mainstream opinion. "People just need to be educated", she said. I am sure **Rose** is correct, but most people don't want to suffer embarrassment, gossip or negative attitudes while they attempt to educate others.

Grace, a cosmetic saleswoman from Staten Island, chose to keep her facelift a secret from her mother and siblings for a different reason. As a single mom whose erratic work schedule is determined by company needs, she doesn't get a regular weekly paycheck or a significant pension to fall back on in later years. "This lack of financial security is a constant worry to my family. They would be horrified if they knew I took out a loan to get a facelift."

In **Grace's** case it was easy to avoid telling her family because they live some distance apart and only see one another a few times a year. By keeping her surgery a secret, she was not only protecting her mother and brother from worry, but also avoiding probable family dissension.

Lauren explained that she is a very private person in general and didn't want people to know, but preferred that they continue to think that she was aging well. She only told her children, sister and husband; but planned her surgery so her husband wouldn't see her immediately post-op.

> "I remarried a few years ago and I wanted to keep the romance alive, so I had my surgery in another city and stayed in a hotel for about two weeks until I felt comfortable to come home to him and look somewhat normal."

She said she was glad she handled it that way.

126

There is another interesting phenomenon about women, secrecy and cosmetic surgery. Many who are secretive about their surgeries readily admit to 'having their eyes done'. **Jennifer** told the story of a friend who had upper and lower eyelifts, yet when she talks about others who have had cosmetic surgery, she doesn't include herself in this group.

"She has a kind of elitist attitude because she didn't have *real* cosmetic surgery. She acts like eyes don't count so she gets special dispensation."

Katherine told her boyfriend she was having her eyes done, when in fact she had a full facelift. She couldn't explain why she didn't mind telling him about her eyes, yet didn't want to admit to all the rest. When he asked her why she had stitches behind her ears, she answered, "Oh, I don't know, I guess that's the way they do eyes now", then laughed aloud as she explained to me: "Men are so stupid. He just accepted that as fact."

As far as secrecy, I think **Nicole** mirrored the feelings many of us experience with time.

> "I was more concerned about what other people thought right after I had the surgery than I am now. Since it has been well over six years since my breast augmentation, I don't care too much how other people react. I look good and feel good and that is all that matters."

But in general, the women I interviewed who remained mute about their surgeries didn't want to deal with judgmental attitudes, criticism, gossip or jealousy. Some were embarrassed or fearful others would think of them as vain, shallow or frivolous. Some wanted others to think of them as younger, including those who believed a more youthful appearance would benefit their careers.

Inventive Deceptions

Do you tell? If not, how do you explain your absence from work, your sudden lack of circulation, your inability to fulfill routine obligations, your bruises and swelling, and finally, your new improved appearance? The number of women opting for full disclose continues to grow, but if you choose to keep your cosmetic surgery a secret, that is your option. You owe no one full disclosure.

Grace, the saleswoman from Staten Island, told me that when her brother's girlfriend repeatedly asked, "What kind of work has your sister had done on her face?" and despite his denials, persisted with the words: "No one looks that good at her age without some surgery', he convinced her otherwise by saying: "Not Grace, we just have good genes in our family." Although he truly believed his own explanation, this line works well for people you newly meet or for those you don't see very often.

Fran Orgovan, the esthetician you already met in Chapter 3, *What Can You Expect After Cosmetic Surgery,* passes along another idea to keep that deception alive.

> "I worked with one plastic surgeon whose patient list included many models and celebrity personalities. I often heard him advise them to change their hairstyle or hair color shortly before facial surgery. People will generally attribute your enhanced appearance to a difference in your hair."

But if people continue to ask, you need to be prepared with some plausible explanation. Here are a few of the most inventive deceptions I have heard:

"What happened to you?" (While healing from a facelift):

"I had the most frightening experience last weekend. A dog darted out in front of my car and I had to swerve sharply to avoid hitting him. Luckily there was no damage to my car, but my airbag just exploded in my face. I always thought there had to be direct impact for an airbag to open."

"I was carrying a box of canned peaches to my downstairs pantry, was so busy trying to balance the box that I didn't pay attention to my feet, tripped and fell down the basement steps. You think this is bad? You should have seen me two days ago."

"What ever happened to you?" (While healing from a nose job):

"I got a horrendous sinus infection. My doctor had to do so much poking to clean out my sinuses that I ended up as bruised as an over ripe peach."

"I got hit by my partner's racket on the tennis courts. My nose was broken, but the doctor says it's healing nicely."

"You look fantastic! What did you do?" (After your facelift has healed):

"My Parisian girlfriend sent me the most marvelous new skin care products. Thanks so much for your great feedback. She said they are hard to come by, but now I definitely will have to beg her to try to get me some more."

"My hair stylist kept coaxing me to let my hair grow so that she could try something altogether different. I finally listened. I'm so glad you like it. "

Because hair is so visible, others are likely to attribute your refreshed appearance to a flattering new hair color or style.

"You look fantastic! What did you do?" (After body sculpting):

> "I finally went on . . . (substitute any diet name of your choice) and began the . . . (substitute any exercise program name of your choice) exercise program. It's really made quite a difference. I'm thrilled. You should try it too."

"Wow! When did you get such a sexy figure?" (After breast augmentation):

> "My doctor put me on medication to regulate my periods (to lessen my hot flahes, etc.) It sure blew up my breasts like two balloons!"

> "My mom told me the same thing happened to her. When she got married, she was a size AA cup, but by the time she turned 30 (40, 50 – you name it) she was a size D. I guess the women in our family are late bloomers."

If you opt for deception, have fun with it. Make up an outrageous story, tell it with conviction (even practice before a mirror beforehand) and you will be likely to convince even the most diehard skeptic.

I received this message from **Arlene**, a former colleague and friend, shortly after she had relocated to South Carolina:

> "I've thought about your note and the reluctance of women to share their experience of surgery. Here's my premise. I remember about ten years ago when I began menopause, few women were willing to talk about symptoms or feel comfortable about admitting they were having flashes, etc. One can't imagine this now because the Boomers have made discussions and

mentions of menopause acceptable in all venues. I think perhaps you are facing a wall that will soon be crumbling. We Pre-Boomers, who were teens in the fifties, seem to have a reserve that our younger sisters lack."

Val tells me that in the past three to four years, she has noticed a big difference in women's willingness to talk about their cosmetic surgeries.

"This is most evident amongst my younger clients, those in the twenty to forty year age range, who are not embarrassed at all. They just talk about it. Perhaps they talk to me more freely because I'm a stylist and sometimes I need to bring this up in reference to their hair; but my older clients, those over fifty, tend to whisper. They're just not comfortable talking about it."

Judith, a retired Special Education teacher from Manhattan, concurs, and compared today's more open attitude toward cosmetic surgery to current acceptance of meeting dates over the Internet. "Years ago very few people did that, but today it's commonplace and an accepted means of meeting people. We just live with much less secrecy in our lives."

Before we move away from the topic of secrecy, **Denise** asked if she could add a word about another type of deceit.

"Sometimes a woman asks her friends if they think she needs cosmetic surgery. If you ask a friend, 'Do I need a facelift?' it's a little like asking, 'Do I look fat in this dress?' Some friends want to reassure you, stroke your ego. Others are just fearful of losing their relationship with you as they know it. You're smart. You're not blind. If you think you look fat in that dress, don't buy it. If you think you need cosmetic surgery, you should probably do it, or at least get some objective, professional advice."

Lies

♪   When you're smilin' . . . keep on smiling   ♪
The whole world smiles with you . . . ♪

Louis Armstrong sang those lyrics with such heart, that he
made us want to believe. But the unvarnished truth is that
after your cosmetic surgery some of your world of family
and friends will smile with you, but others will not. **Denise**
understands that only too well because, from her experience,
she sees that some bonds are strengthened while others are
weakened. Many of your friends and family members will be
happy for you, but if you have the expectation that everyone
will respond with enthusiasm, get ready to alter those
expectations. Denise tells how some spouses and friends get
jealous or feel uncomfortable because this woman they
thought they knew so well seems altered, suddenly looks so
beautiful, exudes happiness, has a new outlook in her life.
Denise explains this transition as the difference between
china on linen and paper plates:

> "When a woman is aware of her new found
> attractiveness, she isn't going to let it sit idle; but
> sometimes friends and family members are taken off
> guard. Think of a person who enters a house and sits
> down at a table set with fine china on beautiful linen.
> She just responds differently than if she ate off of
> paper plates with plastic forks. The comfort level has
> been raised."

Nicole, the young mother from Florida who has appeared
before the FDA in support of women's right to choose breast
augmentation, discovered that for her, the comfort level had
not been raised equally for both sexes.

> "Both men and women notice but their reactions are
> different. Women sometimes seem resentful with an
> attitude like: *Now I have to compete with this?* or *Is*

she that lucky? Are they real? because I'm thin and a C cup is generous for my build. Men notice and enjoy what they see."

Clinical psychologist, **Rose**, said that even her own sister, who is a nurse and absolutely stunning says, "I can't believe you put bacteria (Botox) in your face." Then she laughs and says, "But I smoke cigarettes, so I guess we each pick our own poison." In this case, her sister's comment comes more from genuine concern for **Rose's** well being than negative, judgmental attitudes. But family members can be quite judgmental.

When **Nicole** told her parents she was going to have augmentation surgery, her father's immediate reaction was: "Why does John want you to do this?" He just jumped to the conclusion that this was her husband's need, not hers. Think back to *Chapter 8: What Deters Us*, where I recorded my invented conversation with my own dad, and recall his comment: "Isn't Kenny happy with you the way you are? What are you trying to do? Look for a new boyfriend at this stage of your life?" When it comes to attitudes concerning their daughters' virtue, fathers can be extremely protective in their efforts to keep virtue intact.

Sisters often present a different set of problems, but I suspect much is a reflection of the long term history of their relationship. In **Rose's** case, her sister's reaction was generated by genuine concern tinged with misguided beliefs. **Marilyn**, a college level law professor, told me she hasn't told her two older sisters because she knows exactly what their reactions would be. "They would be very jealous and wouldn't compliment me, but instead would say something negative like that it was a ridiculous waste of money." **Marilyn** hasn't seen them yet, but said, "If they ask me, I will tell them, but I have a 'no ask, no tell' philosophy."

Katherine, the young woman who admitted to having her eyes done, but was reluctant to speak about her facelift, did careful research before selecting her plastic surgeon and felt confidant that she would get a good result. She chose not to discuss her decision with her sister because she knew she would "only get a lecture from her". But the night before her surgery, she did call her sister to avoid hurting her feelings. As **Katherine** explained:

> "True to form, my sister called me back within minutes with some last minute advice about what I should and shouldn't let my surgeon do. Even though I am a mature, intelligent woman, she has never let go of that bossy attitude toward me."

Katherine spoke about how much that phone call unsettled her at a time when she needed to remain calm and confident.

Negative attitudes about cosmetic surgery are sometimes handled with denial. **Jane,** the high school administrator from the suburbs of Chicago, went to a gathering shortly after her own surgery, even though she wasn't completely healed, because she wanted to be with family for the holidays.

> "Do you know that no one said a single word about my surgery. They all pretended that it had never happened. Wouldn't you think they would say something to acknowledge it?"

When she finally told her mother-in-law that she felt hurt that no one mentioned a thing about how she looked after her surgery, her mother-in-law just shrugged her shoulders and said, 'Why should anyone talk about that?'

Jane gave a second example of denial regarding cosmetic surgery. Her niece had a rhinoplasty (nose job) when she was a teenager. After **Jane's** facelift, she told her niece what a good job she felt that plastic surgeon had done on her nose.

"My sister-in-law was irate. She thought it was terrible that I had talked about her daughter's surgery. She said there was never anything wrong with her daughter's nose until she had fallen as a child and injured it. It had been a perfect nose until that fall."

Jane said that her sister-in-law is an educated woman with an MD degree, but that she and the rest of the family act like any kind of cosmetic surgery is something shameful.

What about reactions from friends?

Paula, a former preschool teacher who now owns a Bed and Breakfast, first explained that her right eye had always been larger, and her right eyebrow somewhat higher than those same left-side-of-face features. Her surgeon was able to correct the mismatch to some degree during surgery. No one ever seemed to notice before, but after her facelift she received a strange reactions from one of her friends. Here is **Paula's** story:

"One of my friends had the strangest reaction after my surgery. She did the appropriate things: sent flowers and called to see how I was doing. But the first time she saw me after my surgery, she looked at me and made absolutely no comment. Her husband hugged me a few times and kept telling me how fabulous I looked. My friend said nothing. The next time I saw her she said, 'Now I'm going to be absolutely honest. Your surgeon didn't do a good job on your eyes. They are so uneven.' That was it – absolutely no positive comment."

Paula spoke about how she really needed support and confirmation from her friends after surgery and found this friend's reaction so hurtful. She wondered if she was jealous, but then noticed something interesting. Her friend started to take a real interest in her skin, and her face took on such a lovely glow. Then she joined weight watchers and an exercise class and trimmed down so nicely. **Paula** said she kept encouraging her friend with compliments. Last year this same woman had a facelift.

> "In the long term, I guess it was good that I told her my secret because it helped her take some positive steps for herself. But in the short term, her reaction was really hurtful to me."

What about boy friends and spouses? **Denise** spoke about two of her clients who were in fragile marriages, both of which dissolved after their surgeries. Her first story was about **Alisa**, the forty-seven year old Colorado native who spent years in an unhealthy relationship with a partner who literally held her prisoner. For many years she endured his abuse, lacking the self-confidence to move forward.

When **Alisa** finally recognized that she didn't want to spend the rest of her life in bondage, she made the decision to take charge. She lost sixty pounds, had breast and thigh lifts and a mini tummy tuck to get rid of the excess skin. Then she shed her abusive husband. **Denise** concluded with this happy ending: "After her surgery and divorce, **Alisa** has come out of her shell, looks just beautiful, no longer feels entrapped in the wrong person's body. But most important, she tells me she can't remember ever feeling quite so happy."

Denise's second altered relationship story was about a client named **Laura**, who had been married to the same man for over twenty years, but during the last six of those years there had been no physical intimacy between them. **Laura** filed for divorce the year after her cosmetic surgery and **Denise** reports that she is in a new relationship and is positively glowing – so much so that, "it is obvious she has recaptured what had been missing from her life".

Anne, the Registered Nurse from Harrisburg, Pa., concurred by sharing her surgeon's observations about post cosmetic surgery impacts on some marriages.

"My surgeon told me that after cosmetic surgery, some of his female patients leave their husbands for younger men. That's not me, but I thought it was an interesting comment."

Barbara discovered that her boyfriend became hostile.

> "After my surgery, my boy friend got so snippy toward me. He would lash out at me for little or no reason and was continually questioning my fidelity. I think it has made him feel scared and insecure."

In an article that appeared in a British publication, **Dawn** told how after the birth of her third child, she just hid away in baggy T-shirts and barely went out. Her dress size expanded from a size 10 to a 16 and her abdomen was huge. When her mom offered to treat her to a tummy tuck and liposuction, her husband balked and said, "You're not going." But she was determined and went ahead with the surgery. Even her husband agreed that she looked great afterwards, but it was the final unraveling of their marriage. "It seems there wasn't room in our marriage for my new found confidence. But I have no regrets. It's his loss." **1**

Alice spoke of the mixed messages she has gotten from her spouse. "My husband thinks all this 'beauty stuff' is ridiculous, but then he turns around and tells me that his sister-in-law is aging terribly."

She confided that she thinks he is just insecure about the fact that she looks so good and is getting so much positive attention, but said she did surgery totally for herself.

Fran Orgovan, the esthetician who had recommended that women change their hair color or style before cosmetic surgery, shared something else she has learned from her clients - that generally children don't like their mothers to have cosmetic surgery.

"Daughters often fear losing their mothers, whereas sons don't want their mothers to get more sexual. My own daughter, who is a nurse, called me the day before my surgery to try to dissuade me. She had had a really bad dream the previous night and had become extremely nervous."

During one of our telephone interview sessions, **Fran's** son, **Justin,** walked into the room. She asked him if he'd like to share his feelings about cosmetic surgery. Here are his thoughts:

> "Well, first of all, I want to go to college and I'm afraid there won't be enough money left for me. As far as age, I think you should just get over with it. You are going to get older sooner or later – why don't you just face reality?"

Jean Posillico, a Registered Nurse and clinical esthetician whom you will meet in Chapter 10, *Misperceptions and Misconceptions,* has a sixteen year old son named **Alex.** He told me that when his mom first got started with "this cosmetic stuff", it took him off guard:

> "At first I found it kind of shocking, but now I feel glad for her. After Mom had her eyes done, I could see that it made her so happy. I could see a change in her self-confidence. Afterwards, when she would speak to people, she just seemed more alive."

What an observant young man!

Former fashion model, **Zena,** talked about how she had scheduled surgery while her teenage daughter was away visiting her grandparents. She told her daughter she was having a facelift, but thought it might be frightening for her to see her mom in the early days after surgery.

> "Do you know that when my daughter came back home, she never said a word to me about how I

looked? For some reason, she doesn't want to acknowledge it."

Zena knows that it isn't a matter of forgetting. "My daughter was right in the room when one of my friends was speaking about how great I look. I feel bewildered and hurt by her attitude."

Winnie, a retired social worker from Long Island, has three grown children who live quite a distance from the home they once knew, and consequently she doesn't see them too frequently. Although they were raised without family secrets and encouraged to share openly, **Winnie** did not tell her children of either of her impending surgeries, simply because she didn't want to worry them in advance. After her breast reduction, she was surprised that none of her children commented, because according to **Winnie,** "There was no way they wouldn't have noticed." Then she told this story as a way of further explanation:

> "One day, while visiting my son and daughter-in-law, and sitting around their pool in a bathing suit, I finally asked: 'Don't you notice anything different about me?' My daughter-in-law took another look and said: 'Oh, what did you do? I thought maybe you did something.'"

Six weeks after her facelift **Winnie** drove to New Hampshire to welcome her newest grandchild. Again, none of her children commented, even after the maternity ward nurse said: "Your mother looks so young, I can't believe this is her seventh grandchild."

I speculated that perhaps Winnie's children observed differences in their mother's appearance but didn't comment because she had never spoken to them directly about either of her cosmetic enhancements. But Winnie had a different theory:

"I think they just see Mom as she always was and with the time lapse between our meetings, they just don't see me aging. I know they are very much 'into their own lives' and Mom is just Mom, but I don't mean that in a negative way. They are loving, wonderful people. It's just that they live so far from us that it's not possible to be part of each others' lives on a regular basis."

Whitney, that delightful woman from Cincinnati, Ohio who just happens to be my granddaughter Emily's other grandmother, had a small amount of cosmetic surgery, but would like to have more.

> "My boys, in particular, think that I am crazy whenever I say that if I ever win the lottery, I will include cosmetic surgery on my list of interests. They believe I should be satisfied to grow old gracefully and wrinkled."

In talking about her grown sons, **Carol**, the retired math teacher whose feet never seem to touch the ground, said her three sons felt that she didn't need surgery. "They always thought I was good enough. But when I had it done they were supportive. My second son always tells me how beautiful I look. The other two don't comment."

Lauren, the interior designer from Atlanta, spoke about the reactions from her three children. She received support from all of them, despite general feelings of disapproval.

> "My daughter helped me afterwards, even though she and my older son are more naturalists and don't think we should be tampering with mother nature. My younger son doesn't like change and liked me just the way I was, but he never directly indicated disapproval. I can read between the lines only because I know him so well and understands how he thinks. I discovered that it's possible for a child to

privately disapprove while showing unconditional love and support."

If your son or daughter shows enthusiasm and support for your cosmetic surgery, consider it a real bonus; but don't anticipate that you will get it or feel despondent if you do not, because children generally like the status quo to be maintained.

Not everyone will celebrate your improved appearance. It is possible, though unlikely, that you might not celebrate it yourself. But as we have seen in Chapter 4, *Preferential Treatment for the Pretty Ones*, we can't simply dismiss the importance of appearance with truisms such as: *Appearance doesn't matter, it's what's inside that counts.* For feeling better about yourself can lead to a better life. But not always.

Are the Benefits to Cosmetic Surgery Universal?

The media would make us believe that every person derives untold benefits from cosmetic surgery. Despite all the press and positive post surgery reactions, you need to know that cosmetic surgery is not always the best solution. If you are experiencing other conflicts in your life, you need to resolve them. Don't count on cosmetic surgery to fix all of life's ills. It was never intended as an analgesic and will not make your troubles magically disappear. **Fran Orgovan**, one of our esthetician friends, has observed that women who are basically insecure, shy, inhibited or very focused on the exterior, never seem to be satisfied.

> "I know one woman who had breast augmentation surgery; loves having larger breasts, but it hasn't seemed to have changed her basic insecurity. I suspect that even with a million surgeries, this woman's confidence level wouldn't change."

Some women become more depressed because cosmetic surgery hasn't resolved their inner problems. We are living in a world flooded by images, ruled by consumerism; so it is easy to be lulled into believing that cosmetic surgery will cure whatever ails us, make our troubles drift away, help us discover our inner identities. It will not. Such expectations set us up for future disappointment, even depression. That is why it is best to sort out your expectations before you make this important decision for yourself.

Helpful Resources

See also the following end-of-book helpful resources pertinent to information found in this chapter.

CD Part C: Quiz - Are You a Good Candidate for Cosmetic Surgery

CD Part D: Checklist – Common Signs of Depression

Appendix 8:Personal Profiles
(More about the people whose names appear in this chapter)

Appendix 9: Additional Stories for Chapter 9

Footnotes

1. Carroll, Helen. <u>Mirror.co.uk.</u> "Plastic surgery wrecked our relationship". (2/26/05).

Chapter 10: Misperceptions and Misconceptions

The Short Story:
Correcting common misunderstandings about plastic surgery

"Misperception: A mental grasp based on faulty intuition or insight"

"Misconception: A misunderstanding"

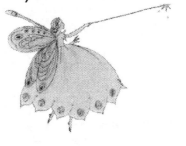

Misperceptions

In an article that appeared in AARP Magazine, Anne Roiphe described glamour as the "flash of excitement across a person's face, . . . the pleasure one takes in life." **1**

Surely she is right: a joyous attitude, an enthusiasm for others and for life's experiences creates an unmistakable aura of attractiveness, perhaps even glamour. But her next sentence: "Plastic surgery can in fact ruin your glamour, causing your face to look like a mask, spoiling your smile, freezing the flash of sympathy and intelligence that used to ripple through your sags and wrinkles", is one that needs clarification.

Yes, plastic surgery can do these things, but it should not and need not. It is all in the hands of the surgeon you choose. The belief that facelifts result in stiff, artificial facial expressions is a misperception based on observations of poor quality surgery or remembrances of facelifts of the not-so-distant past and reinforced by its very name, *plastic* surgery, a word which conjures up visions of that *wind tunnel* look Anne Roiphe described above. In actuality, the name *plastic* surgery was not meant to summon images of the hardened commercial compounds we associate with plastics, but derives from the Greek word 'plastikos', which means to mold or take form. If only the word 'plastikos' had been retained, people would have been more likely to inquire of its meaning rather than jump to faulty conclusions.

A second misperception surrounding cosmetic surgery is that because it's a *cosmetic* procedure, it is less than *real* surgery, and need not be taken as seriously. Certainly, cosmetic surgery is not the same as surgery to repair a damaged heart or kidney, but it is still surgery, and like any elective procedure, should not be undertaken lightly. If you have a medical condition that might complicate your surgical outcome, tread cautiously. Seek consultations with at least two well-qualified plastic surgeons. If they both give you similar cautions about decided risks to your health, don't shop around for a surgeon willing to take those risks. You are likely to find one, but is this really in your best interest?

Even if you are in excellent health and get medical clearance, you still need to anticipate and prepare for a period of recovery. In my Epilogue you will read about **Rosalie** and **Stacey**, the two nurses who monitored my condition, iced my face, fed and medicated me, taught me how to care for my healing body and calmed and entertained me during those first sixteen post surgery hours. Yet before my surgery, I debated the need for a post surgery nurse, as I was still under the misperception that: "After all, I'm healthy and there is

146

nothing medically wrong with me, so I really don't need a nurse." I was wrong.

In her early days of healing, **Lauren**, the interior designer from Atlanta, discovered that an experienced cosmetic surgery nurse is somewhat akin to a guardian angel. Here is her story:

> "The nurse who accompanied me back to the hotel was okay, but the nurse who came the next day was incredible. She thought of everything. I had trouble opening my mouth far enough to brush my teeth with a regular toothbrush, but my wonderful nurse went out and bought me a baby Oral B toothbrush that worked really well. She taught me how to spit out of a straw when brushing my teeth. I know this sounds strange, but this was a really useful skill to learn. As you know, you are not supposed to bend your head back and forth too much after a facelift, but it is almost impossible to brush, rinse and spit without bending your head. That straw made such a difference.'

> "At first I also had trouble eating some types of food. My wonderful nurse made me soft foods like oatmeal and liquids like thin soups that I could drink with a straw. She fixed me toast with honey and jelly and cut it into little strips that made it manageable. And did I tell you she gave me a foot massage at 3:00 AM? She was so amazing. She thought of everything that could improve my comfort level.'

> "I think it is so important to have a caring, capable nurse with you for the first 24-48 hours. There are so many questions and concerns that can be put to rest by a compassionate, experienced professional."

An adjunct to that misperception that cosmetic surgery is not *real* surgery, is the attitude that you are foolish to be nervous. Some of us will be nervous no matter what. When you read my Epilogue, you will learn that I certainly was, but you will also discover two effective visualization strategies I used to help calm myself.

Don't necessarily anticipate that you will get last minute jitters, but on the other hand, know that you're not alone if you do. Be sure to read some of the additional stories about other women's varied states of pre-surgery composure - or lack thereof - in Appendix 9 at the back of this book. The stories from both **Denise Thomas** and the other women I interviewed offer some important implications worth considering:

Implication 1: Select your surgeon with utmost care and then place your faith and trust in him.

Implications 2: Once you feel confidence in your doctor, remain focused on the positive result he will achieve for you.

Implication 3: Don't try to orchestrate the surgery. You have already told your doctor what you want. Now trust him and his judgment to do the best job he possibly can. On the other hand, if you previously made a special request that you think your surgeon might be likely to overlook, such as that mole on your chin or stretch mark on your abdomen, write a note as a reminder. Before you are sedated, ask the nurse or other attending medical staff member to please pass this note along to your surgeon before he enters the O.R.

Implication 4: Prior to your surgery, you might want to ask your surgeon if you can speak with one or two of his patients who have undergone similar procedures. If possible, try to arrange to meet with them to see their surgical results. **Denise** often introduces pre-surgery clients to other of her clients who have already undergone similar procedures with the same surgeon, and finds that that contact gives them just the right touch of reassurance they need.

Implication 5: Avoid situations that might unnerve you. When you read **Jane's** story in Appendix 9, notice how she turned down her husband's offer to drive her to her surgery, but made alternative arrangements to prevent his nervousness from spilling over onto her.

Implication 6: If cosmetic surgery can fix something about your face or body that continually undermines your self-esteem and there are no serious contra indications for surgery, go for it. After you read **Jean** and **Nicole's** stories in Appendix 9, you will be reassured that you are worth it.

Implication 7: If you think you might become unduly nervous, consider asking your doctor for a prescription to calm your nerves, but *do not take anything without your doctor's approval*. **Norma Jean** and **Lauren** both obtained prescriptions from their surgeons and found that those prescribed substances helped them relax.

Implication 8: Select one good friend or close relative to serve as your support system, to be with you before surgery and in your early post-operative days. Do something you enjoy with your special support person on the day/evening before your surgery. In Appendix 9, **Maria** shares a great story about her special support buddy and the wedding they attended the night before her surgery.

Implication 9: Educate yourself in advance about the procedure(s) you are considering. Appendix 6 at the back of this book gives you some helpful resources. Most of us are calmed by getting the facts. This knowledge helps you ask more intelligent questions and more readily understand the answers you are given. **Anne's** knowledge of her forthcoming procedures and familiarity with the facility where her surgery would take place gave her confidence and a sense of calm.

The third set of misperceptions about cosmetic surgery relate to concerns about post surgery pain and erratic surgical result. Yet my personal experiences, as well as those of most women I interviewed, spoke in terms of moderate, well controlled discomfort and high levels of satisfaction with their ultimate results.

When I asked women to describe their recovery in terms of healing time and pain, many shared stories similar to those of **'Makeover'**, **'Sunshine'**, **Hope**, **'Realtor'** and **Jane** who described the discomfort they experienced as less than or equal to their expectations and said they healed without incident. **Norma Jean**, another Questionnaire Respondent, as well as interview subjects **Marilyn**, the college law professor, and hairstylist, **Val**, were all on painkillers for a number of days after their surgeries, which kept them comfortable. Their biggest voiced complaint about painkillers was their annoying side effect of constipation. Some discovered that they needed to take stool softeners to ease a problem that **Val** described as "nearly as bad as childbirth".

There are many variables involved in the healing process and it would be a mistake for me to leave you with the impression that post surgery healing always goes totally without incident. All of the women I interviewed had selected experienced, board certified plastic surgeons, and even so, a few of them described bumpy roads in their recoveries. But ultimately each of them was highly satisfied with her surgical results. And that is the bottom line. Those who selected their surgeons wisely ultimately had good results.

I asked several women who experienced temporary healing difficulties to share their personal words of wisdom. I wanted you to listen to their stories, not to frighten you, but to help you focus on that proverbial light at the end of the tunnel.

Lauren, the interior designer from Atlanta, never complained about pain, but said she was totally unprepared for the swelling she experienced after her facelift. "I remember looking in the mirror and not recognizing the person staring back at me." She said that before her surgery, most people would have considered her most attractive. But for the first several post surgery days, all she could see was a very unattractive woman and she wondered if she would ever look the same.

> "I felt sadness. I had never felt ugly before. Every day I would look in the mirror, hoping to see a glimpse of my old self and kept wondering: *What have I done? Will I ever be the same?* I felt guilt because I had elected to have these procedures done to myself and knew that there were people such as burn or accident victims, who never elected to have changes made to their bodies, who sometimes had to live with those altered appearances forever."

Now that **Lauren** is fully recovered and so happy with the results of her facelift, she wants to tell other women to "exercise lots and lots of patience and don't expect to be healed and seeing the finished product too soon. Understand it's a process and healing continues long after we think we're done."

Law professor, **Marilyn**, described the tightness she felt under her chin and around her neck as "areas that felt like they were bound with restrictive tape that I wished I could peel off." She was told this feeling would gradually lessen for up to one year, but said that she wasn't big on the delayed gratification part of this process. **Marilyn's** words of advice are similar to those **Lauren** gave above: "Don't expect immediate results or instant gratification. Healing has its own schedule."

Nicole, the woman who appeared before the FDA in support of a woman's right to choose breast augmentation, echoed their thoughts; "Know that time is your best friend. Be patient."

Fran Orgovan, the esthetician whose hobby is painting nudes, explained why some depression or crashing might occur two or three days after surgery:

> "Anesthesiologists often infuse the patient through their IV at the end of surgery. They use a steroid called Decadron to reduce swelling, but it tends to bring the body up emotionally as well. Know that as it wears off, you might crash a bit and feel some depression."

I asked **Fran** if there were ways that she was able to help herself during recovery. Were there any proactive steps she took for herself or advises her clients to take to bolster their morale?

> "Camouflage the after effects of your new surgery while healing so that you can be around other people as soon as possible.", **Fran** advised. "Then ask a nurse or esthetician to show you how to apply concealing make-up. You can use concealer to hide facial bruises, wear a scarf around your neck to conceal swelling. The worst thing for your morale is to hide away in the house."

Fran encourages her clients to discuss their post surgery feelings, because once they discover that they are not alone, they feel reassured. She also instructs them on how to massage properly around their eyes and other surgical sites. She suggests that all patients get instruction on massage from a nurse or esthetician during their early post surgery days, because massage helps the healing process.

Jean Posillico, a registered nurse/esthetician, cautioned that we all heal differently and that sometimes complications occur which slow down that process.

"When complications do occur, it is all too common to point blame, which is counter productive to a healthy mental outlook. Understand that this is your defense mechanism kicking in and that you will help yourself if you avoid this unnecessary negativity. Instead, you can help your body heal by learning how to massage the surgical site to bring oxygenated blood to the area."

Jean speaks from personal experience. After her breast reduction surgery, she developed a pooling of blood in one breast, a condition known in medical terms as a hematoma. The swelling from this hematoma put pressure on her stitches, causing them to open prematurely. After her stitches opened, that one breast healed more slowly. **Jean** explained that for women, breasts are an anatomical feature that often defines them. Initially, when she saw the unhealed scar on her one breast, she became depressed. She knew that her husband didn't want her to have breast reduction surgery, and was reluctant to even take off her blouse and show him her scarred body. She felt like she had made a terrible mistake. But eight weeks later, when she no longer had any pain and could see cosmetic improvement daily, she began to realize that this surgery would be 'life altering' for her.

Because of **Jean's** complication, she needed to postpone her scheduled return to work by a full week, a situation that heightened her feelings of depression and isolation. She mirrored some of **Fran's** thoughts when she said: "It is important to get out of the house and be with other people as soon as you feel physically able to do so. I know I felt so much better as soon as I got back to work."

Later in this chapter, as you read about **Jean's** history with medications and her recommendation for those of you who have been on certain medicines long term, you will learn why it is crucial to reveal *everything* about your health and health habits to your surgeon. No matter how competent he is, you must also assume some of the responsibility for a successful outcome.

Nicole spoke about how she and her surgeon had made the decision to place her implants beneath her chest muscles, which were very tight due to all her weight training. Unlike many of the women in her breast augmentation support groups, who experience little pain and are almost back to themselves several days after surgery, **Nicole's** breasts were both hard and sore for about three months before they gradually became softer with a more natural feel. She spoke about how, for the first year after her surgery, she experienced sensation so heightened that her nipples would stand out from the slightest touch and required the use of cotton pads to soothe them. Because of her slow recovery, **Nicole** went through some depression, but, as you already know from her other stories throughout this book, **Nicole's** surgical results have been professionally and personally life altering.

Nicole reminds women not to be embarrassed to discuss their concerns with their doctors. For example, she frequently sees women's postings about loss of breast sensation on her Internet Discussion Board.

> "This is a topic they often feel embarrassed to discuss with their surgeons. Remember, your surgeon is not a mind reader. You need to tell him your thoughts before he can respond to them."

She also reminds women that they can get support from other sources. "There are support groups you can join as well as on-line discussion groups where you can speak with other women willing to share their experiences."

Misconceptions

Because of certain gray areas in this field, your safety and ultimately your life may depend upon your choice of surgeon. Yet in the official medical journal of the American Society of Plastic Surgeons, ASPS Past-President, Rod Rohrich, MD, claims that people rarely do their research.

> *In America, most people spend more time finding the right pair of shoes than they do finding a cosmetic plastic surgeon. You can take back your shoes, but you can't take your face or your life back.* **3**

Here are the facts to clear up a few misconceptions:

Any licensed physician, regardless of training, can legally perform plastic surgery and call himself a plastic or cosmetic surgeon.
Would you want a board certified gynecologist or allergist to perform your cosmetic surgery? Of course not! But although only a handful of the twenty-four medical specialties recognized by the American Board of Medical Specialties (ABMS) include any surgical training, legally any board certified physician is permitted to perform your cosmetic surgery.

Managed care has ushered in some undesirable changes to the practice of medicine, including the rush of physicians from diverse specialties to suddenly transform themselves into plastic surgeons. Their motivation is clear: to bypass the managed care system and deal directly with the patient and her checkbook. Make no mistake about it, plastic surgery is a *surgical* specialty. Treat it as such. Don't call in a plumber to fix your electrical wiring!

Official sounding titles are not always legitimate.
There are only twenty-four medical specialty boards recognized by the American Board of Medical Specialties (ABMS). Yet over one hundred thirty board names, each

carrying an official sounding title, appear in advertisements, on physician websites and more. Be aware that some of these boards are self-appointed, while others are simply bogus. Each of them carries an official sounding title, beginning with the words: "American Board of . . ." . The insertion of even one additional word into a highly respected board title can spell the difference between a skilled surgeon with seven years of specialized training and one who has taken a few weekend courses of additional training. Beware those title nuances.

If you see the words: American Board of *Cosmetic* Surgery or American Board of *Facial* Surgery as part of a board title under a doctor's name, put on your running shoes and sprint in the opposite direction. There is no board recognized by the American Board of Medical Specialties (ABMS) with the word *cosmetic* or *facial* in its title, yet at least eight different boards exist with titles that include one of those words. Another deceptive ploy is to use only the words *Board Certified*. You want to be sure your surgeon is board certified by the *American Board of Medical Specialties*.

Several board specialties are certified by the American Board of Medical Specialties (ABMS) to perform cosmetic surgery. How do you choose? Members of the American Board of Plastic Surgery and the American Board of Otolaryngology - that is, both the board certified plastic surgeon and the board certified otolaryngologist (aka head and neck surgeons or ENT specialists) - have completed a minimum of five years of postgraduate surgical training. The difference lies in the scope of their training. Whereas the otolaryngologist is certified to perform head and neck surgeries only, the plastic surgeon is certified to perform surgeries to any part of the face or body.

Additionally, there are board certified ophthalmologists and board certified dermatologists who have had advanced cosmetic surgical training in their respective fields.

If you have a narrowly focused surgical need, (e.g. a cosmetic procedure related to your eyes, your skin, your nose, your neck), a physician from one of these specialties might be a good choice for you. Otherwise select a board certified plastic surgeon.

Ultimately, your choice should depend upon the surgeon's training, experience and expertise, so inquire about all three. Experience counts. Before you consider a surgeon from any of the above specialties, you should know how frequently he performs the specific procedures you are considering. We all hone our skills through repetition. Surgeons, who continue to fine tune their skills and surgical judgment with experience, are no exception. That is why it is important that you select someone with not only the proper credentials, but who also **a)** devotes most of his practice to *cosmetic* surgical procedures and **b)** has done the procedures which relate to your needs many times and continues to do so on a regular basis. Because facelifts require so much artistry, I would want my surgeon to have done a minimum of one hundred facelifts before doing mine. More would be better.

Is cosmetic surgery safe or am I putting myself at risk?

If you are healthy and work with a well-qualified surgeon, cosmetic surgery rarely places your life at risk. Every activity we undertake portends some degree of risk. The risk to your life from cosmetic surgery is very small, so small that when such a death occurs, it makes big headlines. A total of 2,185,000 cosmetic surgeries were performed in the US in the year 2005. How many times have you read about a cosmetic surgery fatality?

In a study reported in Plastic Reconstructive Surgery evaluating the safety of office surgical facilities, only one death occurred in 58,810 surgical procedures, a statistic comparable to the overall risk for hospital based surgeries. **4** Here is the caveat: All of these procedures were performed in office surgery facilities *accredited* by the AAASF

(American Association for Accreditation of Ambulatory Surgery Facilities), which mandates that each doctor be board certified in the medical specialty recommended for that procedure and that he has been granted hospital privileges to perform those same procedures in a hospital setting. No statistics exist for surgeries performed in non-accredited surgical facilities, but such statistics undoubtedly would present a different picture.)

You can see that it is rare for someone to actually die while undergoing cosmetic surgery in a hospital or *accredited* surgical facility, but very occasionally a death does occur. To put these cosmetic surgery statistics in better perspective, consider the following facts:

According to the U.S. Department of Transportation, in 2004 there were 8.31 female highway fatalities for every 100,000 women drivers between the ages of twenty-one and sixty-four, the gender and age range within which most cosmetic surgeries occur. This is over four times the number of deaths which occurred per 100,000 cosmetic surgery patients.

But highway deaths are relatively commonplace and don't raise the same eyebrows as deaths reported about those seeking beauty.

If you are in good health, have selected a qualified, experienced board certified surgeon, have scheduled your surgery at an *accredited* facility and have followed all your surgeon's instructions carefully; you life is far safer in his operating room than in an automobile. If you are a good candidate for cosmetic surgery and truly want this for yourself, I would advise you to go for the surgery. This is one day you will be off the highway, where you are more prone to a fatality than in an accredited facility with a skilled surgeon and anesthesiologist.

Your surgeon's hospital privileges are still important, even if your surgery will take place in an outside surgical facility. You want a surgeon who has been given privileges at each hospital where he is on staff. You will then know that his performance and credentials have been subjected to regular scrutiny and approval. Here is why: Once a candidate applies for specific hospital privileges, the surgical chief makes a judgment based on the candidate's credentials and specialty training. In some cases or for more challenging procedures, the chief will also observe this candidate's surgical skills. Sometimes a surgeon is granted hospital privileges for only certain procedures and not others.

Be certain your surgeon has been approved to perform the specific procedures you are considering. If a doctor's privileges have been withheld, it indicates that the chief is not yet satisfied with this surgeon's advanced training or some of his surgical skills. You deserve expertise, not a surgical practice session. *Do not allow any physician to perform procedures for which he has not been granted hospital privileges, even if your surgery is to take place in a non-hospital setting.*

Use your phone book or information services to obtain the hospital telephone number. Then request that doctor's *delineation of privileges*, the procedures he is certified to perform at that hospital.

Don't be overly impressed by the physician whose name constantly appears in print or other media. Such exposure is probably more a testament to his PR agent than his skill as a surgeon. Be aware that many names are out there because of a media blitz arranged by the doctor's publicity agent, and as impressive as this publicity may be, it has little to do with the plastic surgeon's skill. To the contrary, the best plastic surgeons rarely advertise. They don't need to. Their reputations do that for them.

It is one thing to be published in a popular magazine, quite another to appear in a peer reviewed journal. When a physician's article is published in a medical journal, his work has been assessed by a jury of his peers. It is considered worthy of publication only if it accurately informs, educates or expands professional knowledge on a given topic. Popular print media base publication decisions on a very different set of criteria, depending on the interest of their particular readership.

Be sure a board certified anesthesiologist is in charge of your anesthesia, even if you will be getting Twilight as opposed to General Anesthesia.

I asked **Marie Gemma**, a Registered Nurse whom you will meet again in my Epilogue, for her thoughts about anesthesia. Here are her words:

> "The person who administers your anesthesia is truly the unsung hero in every Operating Room. Be it Twilight (conscious sedation) or General, he is ultimately responsible for your breathing and your life. If you have a liver or kidney impairment, this is particularly significant because anesthesia can be metabolized by those organs.'

> "Your anesthesiologist has to choose the right anesthesia for your body and then know what to do if your system is not responding properly. Nurse anesthetists are well trained, but they are not physicians and don't have the formal education or the expertise to know how to handle some of the emergencies that can arise. I would only want a board certified anesthesiologist to administer and monitor my anesthesia."

Outside surgical facilities are a safe alternative as long as they are accredited.

According to statistics reported by the American Society for Aesthetic Plastic Surgery (ASAPS), seventy-six percent of cosmetic procedures were performed in office based or free standing surgical facilities in 2005 and only twenty-four percent in hospital settings. The good news is that *accredited* office based facilities have a safety record equal to that of hospital ambulatory surgery settings, and many professionals and patients prefer this setting. The bad news is that only a minority of states within the USA currently have mandated accreditation. Don't assume that any facility is accredited without doing your homework.

Denise Thomas explains her preference for surgeries performed in the physician's own *accredited* ambulatory surgery facility.

> "I want to be assured that the surgeon I select for each of my clients is the surgeon who is present and accountable for all of the surgery and never turns his patient over to another physician for selected tasks."

There are three associations that evaluate and accredit outside surgical facilities. The nation's largest organization for accreditation of office based surgery centers is the AAAASF (American Association for Accreditation of Ambulatory Surgery Facilities, Inc.). If your surgery will take place in a facility accredited by the AAAPS, know that they have already done part of your homework for you, as they only accredit office based facilities where the physician in charge is **a)** board certified in the specialty that relates to the specific procedures he performs and **b)** has hospital privileges to perform those same procedures that he schedules in his office based facility. The other two accrediting associations are the AAAHC (Accreditation Association for Ambulatory Health Care) and JCAHO (Joint Commission on Accreditation of Healthcare Organizations). You should make certain that the facility at which your surgery is expected to take place is accredited by one of these associations.

A number of women have told me that they would feel safer having surgery in a hospital setting "just in case anything happens." At one time I would have agreed, but now that I understand the stringent requirements for accreditation, my preference would be for an accredited outside surgical facility unless I had compromised health that might necessitate an interdisciplinary approach. Accredited sites must be equipped with the same emergency equipment that would be found in a hospital emergency room (e.g. defibrillator, compression board, airway equipment, supplemental oxygen, emergency medications and more) to stabilize a patient-in-crisis. An advanced cardiologist life support trained member must be present during all phases of surgery.

I like the personalized care the patient receives in an *Accredited Surgical Facility*, with fewer distractions for the surgeon and his staff. Furthermore, hospitals carry an additional, not uncommon risk – the transmission of infection – something unlikely to occur in an office based surgery center.

Even though you have complete confidence in your surgeon, some of the responsibility for a successful outcome rests in your hands.
"You must reveal *everything* about your health and health habits to your surgeon", says **Jean Posillico**, the registered nurse/esthetician who developed a hematoma after her breast reduction surgery.

> "Include illnesses and your use of prescriptive, over-the-counter, herbal, habitual and addictive drugs. Many of these substances can conflict with certain forms of anesthesia or cause complications during or after surgery. For example, ordinarily, when people complete those questionnaire forms for their

surgeons, they check off 'light use of alcohol', forgetting that a bottle of wine consumed with dinner is also alcohol. You need to consider all forms of ingestion carefully and answer forthrightly. Be honest with your doctor. Don't hold back anything. Your recovery, sometimes even your life, depend upon your full disclosure."

Although **Jean** is a Registered Nurse who says she 'should have know better', she admits that she felt embarrassed to share facts with her surgeon about her prolonged use of pain relieving medications to help alleviate her chronic back pain.

"I never exceeded the recommended daily dosages on the labels and even though I followed my surgeon's advice and discontinued all medications for ten days prior to surgery, I now feel that this time frame was insufficient. If you are on any medication or herbal remedy long term and in significant doses, any preparation that your physician advises you to discontinue prior to surgery, the customarily recommended ten day abstention period may be insufficient. Once these ingredients get into your blood, it takes a long time for them to dissipate."

Jean believes that the pain relieving medications still in her blood caused her hematoma and that if she had been more forthright with her surgeon, he might have advised her to discontinue their usage earlier - (perhaps four weeks prior to surgery rather than the customary ten days) - to avoid possible complications.

As an end to our discussion about cosmetic surgery and embarrassment, **Jean** spoke about the philosophy she has tried to impart to her children:

"We should never be ashamed of our bodies. If you are unhappy with your body image, do everything you can through diet and exercise. But if that isn't sufficient, know that cosmetic surgery is a viable option."

You have just read many facts to clear up eight common misconceptions. Remember, knowledge gives you the power both to choose wisely and help yourself to a successful outcome. In the words of Robert Bernard, MD, Past-President of the ASAPS (American Society for Aesthetic Plastic Surgery):

The public has to know what questions to ask so that they can make the right decisions about their medical care.

Helpful Resources

See also the following end-of-book helpful resources pertinent to information found in this chapter.

CD Part E: Checklist – Questions to Ask <u>Before</u> a Consultation

CD Part F: Checklist – Questions to Ask <u>During</u> a Consultation

CD Part G: Quiz – Rate Your Reaction to Your Consultation (The Third <u>R</u>)

CD Part H: Timeline Checklists – What to Do and When

Appendix 4: Selecting the Surgeon Who Is Right For You –
(Begin With the Two R's: <u>R</u>eferrals and <u>R</u>esearch)

Appendix 5: Relaxation Techniques – Ways to Calm Your Mind

Appendix 6: Internet and Book Resources

Appendix 7: Associations, Medical Boards, Web-sites and more

☼ **Appendix 8: Personal Profiles**
(More about the people whose
names appear in this chapter)

☼ **Appendix 9: Additional Stories for Chapter 10**

Footnotes

1. Roiphe A. "Glamour". <u>AARP Magazine</u>. (March/April 2003): 38-39.

2. U. S. Department of Transportation's Fatality Analysis <u>http://www.nrd.nhtsa.dot.gov/pdf/nrd-30/nsca/TSF2004.pdf</u>: 104.

3. <u>Plastic and Reconstructive Surgery</u>. (4.27.04).

4. Keyes G. Singer R. Iverson R. McGuire M. Yates J. Gold A. and Thompson D. "Analysis of outpatient surgery center safety using an Internet-based quality improvement and peer review program. <u>Plastic and Reconstructive Surgery</u>. 113.1160 (2004).

Chapter 11: Changing Attitudes: From Freud to the 21ST Century

The Short Story:
Those bad vibes are melting away.

"Vibes: (Colloquial form of the word 'vibrations')
A characteristic emanation, aura or spirit that infuses or
vitalizes someone or something and that can be instinctively
sensed or experienced"

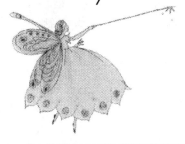

"I have more important things to do with my time than to cater to someone who just cares about her looks."

These are the words a nurse once spoke to her fifteen year old patient, who had just asked for headache medication following otoplasty (surgery to correct prominent ears). This episode, reported in RN Magazine, concluded with the words: What's going on here? Do we, who care so much about most of our patients, discriminate against this one class of patients? If so, it's time we scrutinized the reasons for our behavior."[1]

Even within the medical profession, prejudicial attitudes about cosmetic surgery were alive and well in 1986, the date when this article was written. The stigma surrounding cosmetic surgery has lessened considerably, but has continued to die a slow death. Even today, this event can be shrouded beneath a veil of secrecy. Why should this be?

To uncover the origins of these negative attitudes, we need to look back forty to fifty years, when prevalent thought was slanted toward the psychological instability of the cosmetic surgery patient. It was not uncommon then for researchers to focus on the psychopathology of those seeking cosmetic forms of surgery. Motivations were expressed as a means of warding off depression. Patients were generally characterized as highly neurotic and/or narcissistic, with ambivalent feelings about intimacy and close personal relationships or with fears about aging and abandonment. **2(Hill & Silver) 3(Edgerton, Jacobson & Meyer) 4(Webb, Slaughter, Meyer & Edgerton)**

Sarwer and Crerand have identified three generations of research relating to the cosmetic surgery patient. **5** During that first generation, the period between the 1940's – 1960's, medical journal articles customarily put a Freudian spin on motivations for cosmetic surgery. Some of the earliest interpretations included the symbolic meaning of body parts. Others applied elaborate psychoanalytic interpretations as megalomaniac thinking, latent homosexuality, narcissism, incestuous desires or sadistic behavior as explanations for one's desire for cosmetic surgery. Researchers generally concluded that consultations for reasons other than trauma should be considered an overt symptom of neurosis. One study concluded with the following words:

> ". . . with few exceptions, the patients who presented themselves for rhinoplasty (nose surgery) were ill from a psychiatric point of view. This illness varied from minor neurotic disturbance to overt schizophrenic psychoses." **6**

Although these 'scientifically determined beliefs' were a result of flawed methodologies, once accepted as fact, they were tenaciously endorsed without further questioning. The Freudian view of psychological underpinnings to cosmetic surgery became so entrenched that it was accepted as unquestionable truth. But during that second generation of research, the 1970's – the 1980's, the tenacity of those beliefs had begun to break down.

Researchers introduced more standardized assessment tools, such as the well-validated Minnesota Multiphasic Personality Inventory, to assess personality disorders in cosmetic surgery patients. In three separate relatively small studies they analyzed the personalities of:

a) Fifty facelift patients [7]
b) Ten breast augmentation patients [8]
c) Twenty-five rhinoplasty patients. [9]

In each of these studies, none of the cosmetic surgery patients were found to exhibit any significant psychopathology.

In a fourth, somewhat larger study, one hundred female cosmetic surgery patients were statistically paired with one hundred women specifically assessed as having normal values. Study results indicated that those undergoing cosmetic surgery felt no greater dissatisfaction with their overall appearance than the comparative 'normal value' group. They simply reported substantially greater dissatisfaction with the specific facial or body feature that was being surgically altered. [10]

Psychologists and psychiatrists began to express more accepting attitudes toward those who chose surgery to improve their appearance.

"Those who are relatively unconcerned about their appearance often find it difficult to understand someone's decision to have a facelift, a rhinoplasty, or some other operation which is intended to change and improve appearance. Many believe that a desire to change a surface appearance reflects a superficiality in that person's personality, a vanity, an emptiness, or a self-centered narcissism. They have never thought much about the intimate connection between one's sense of self and one's feelings about one's body." **11**

There was a trickle down effect from those second generation psychological studies, which ushered in an attitude both of greater acceptance of those seeking appearance enhancements through surgery and recognition of the psychological stability of those patients. As first generation psychopathological theories increasingly gave way to theories of psychological normalcy, dissatisfaction with one's appearance, rather than mental illness, became recognized as the principal motivational force behind cosmetic surgery. **12**(Bank), **13**(Maksud & Anderson), **14**(Pruzinsky).

Beyond the research, there were further compelling reasons why the tides continued to shift toward increased acceptance of cosmetic surgery:

• Growing Recognition of the Benefits to Looking Good
As atavistic prejudices and thoughts of trivial vanity began to melt away, they were replaced by attitudes touting the benefits accruing to those undergoing cosmetic surgery:

"Beauty has a known influence on social desirability. Pretty people get better jobs more easily -- studies show they can achieve higher occupational status with less effort -- and their marital prospects are enhanced." **15**

With words simplistic yet wise, my grandfather used to say: "It's easy to love a beautiful person." During that second generation of studies, research continued to document what my grandfather knew all along: Society expresses a bias toward physically attractive people. In Chapter 4, *Preferential Treatment for the Pretty Ones*, you read the results of some of the independent studies regarding the preferential treatment afforded good looking people. One only needs to read through several of these second generation studies to be convinced of my grandfather's wisdom.

> "While dissatisfaction with one's appearance was often dismissed as trivial vanity years ago, (second generation) research has demonstrated the importance of appearance in everyday life. Not only are more physically attractive individuals perceived more favorably than those who are less attractive, it also appears that they receive preferential treatment in interpersonal and social situations. Given this knowledge, improving one's appearance through cosmetic surgery can often be a positive, healthy self-care strategy." **16**

Baby Boomers Debunk the 'Age Gracefully' Philosophy

According to the ASAPS (American Society for Aesthetic Plastic Surgery), last year the Baby Boomers, those born between 1946-64, underwent over half the cosmetic eyelid (bletharoplasty), tummy tuck (adominoplasty) and liposuction (lipoplasty) surgeries performed in the United States. Additionally Baby Boomers are the majority consumer group for those less invasive procedures and treatments often dubbed 'lunchtime procedures' because they fit so well into busy lifestyles. Botox injections, microdermabrasion, soft tissue fillers (e.g. Cosmoderm, Restylane, fat injections), light chemical peels and laser treatments permit one to literally schedule a noon treatment and be back at work in the early afternoon.

With increasing numbers, women today continue to exhibit an unwillingness to buy into that *age gracefully* philosophy and the Baby Boomers have led the parade. Generation Xers, those born between 1965-74, show signs of following in their Boomer sisters' footsteps, predominately with breast augmentation and lipoplasty (liposuction) surgeries, as well as many of the non-surgical pick-me-ups mentioned above.

Increased Life Expectancy and Quality of Life

Life expectancy has risen dramatically in the past century - from an age expectancy of 47 years in 1900 to 77.6 years in 2003. **17** Our era of lengthened life expectancy has nourished new attitudes about aging. As longevity expands for more and more people, so do their expectations for quality of life. Attitudes of maintaining a healthy body and youthful appearance prevail for continually increasing numbers of seniors.

Our seniors are already the fastest growing population group in the USA today. **18, 19** The U.S. Census Bureau reports that as of July, 2005, one in eight people in the United States was age 65 or older, a 33 % increase in five years. The Central Intelligence Agency projects that by the end of 2006, 12.5 % of our population will be age sixty-five or older. Today's Baby Boomers will be the ones sporting Medicare cards within the next decade. As those Medicare eligible numbers continue to soar, it is likely that the number of seniors opting for cosmetic surgery will escalate to new highs.

• Attitudes Within the Medical Profession

This shift in attitude toward cosmetic surgery has become evident within the medical profession as well. A Stanford University trained plastic surgeon anonymously confided to

Denise Thomas that when he chose plastic surgery as his area of specialization, his colleagues criticized him for trying to interfere with God's work. At that time, plastic surgery was generally regarded as a prostitution of science. Today, he describes plastic surgery as a highly respected medical specialty with strong backing from several prestigious medical organizations.

• Improvements in Surgery and Anesthesia

Improvement in surgical and anesthesia techniques has led to simplified surgeries, faster recovery times, decreased risks and far more natural results than in the past, as long as you work with a skilled, well qualified specialist. The many improvements and refinements in cosmetic surgery have encouraged more people to take this step for themselves. *But the competence and experience of the physician are key, so please heed the advice in the second section of Chapter 10, Misperceptions and Misconceptions, with utmost care.*

• Environmental Influences

We are all products of the environment in which we live. Certainly in this 21st century, the profusion of articles, TV shows, commercials and discussions about beauty in general and the benefits of cosmetic surgery in particular bombard us relentlessly. Although the majority of these media images are directed at women, they influence society as a whole. **20**(Monteath & McCabe), **21**(Fredrickson & Robert) **22**(Sarwer).

Are we lured by these societal attitudes? My answer would be an unquestionably yes, I do believe environmental influences are a decided factor furthering growth in cosmetic surgery numbers. The media help shape our identities and our ideologies. We are influenced by the messages that surround us, including the current cosmetic surgery 'media madness'. There is little doubt that the communication media of reality based television, magazines, newspapers and movies continually inundate us with messages designed to heighten standards of beauty.

Mass media influences help shape the trends, most recent of which is the idealized image of a woman. She stands taller, yet weighs less. She is slimmer, yet more muscular. Her breasts are larger. The figure just described is a body type atypical to nature, yet that image fuels expectations and discontent. If we were living on a planet where good looks were not so highly valued, where no extra privileges were bestowed upon better looking people, cosmetic surgery statistics undoubtedly would decline. But instead, we are living in an environment that promotes heightened expectations, probing self-inspections, deeper dissatisfactions and greater investment in appearance.

> "These socio cultural influences shape our interest in appearance enhancing behaviors in many ways. The most direct way is likely through the development of body image dissatisfaction, which in turn is thought to play a central role in the pursuit of cosmetic surgery, as well as many appearance-related pursuits such as weight loss and cosmetic use." **23**

This brings us to the juncture of that third generation of research, begun in the 1990's and still ongoing today. Recent studies on anti-aging, while stating that cosmetic surgery patients are not so psychopathological as determined by early research, note that:

> "Patients seeking anti-aging procedures may place greater emphasis on their appearance, and seek surgery to decrease body image dissatisfaction specifically associated with aging facial features" **24**

Pride in one's appearance is often a reflection of healthy self-esteem, but can be damaging if appearance begins to dictate one's self worth. Because third generation research findings are beginning to suggest an upward trend in body image dissatisfaction, we need to reflect on where we as a society are headed. When NFO WorldGroup, a Greenwich, Connecticut-based market research company surveyed a nationally representative sample of adults, a total of 87% of these men and women said that if they could change any part of their body for cosmetic reasons, they would do so, and half of those same respondents said they would change many body parts. On a scale of 1-10, with one being the lowest, 47% gave themselves a score of five or under when asked how happy they were with their physical appearance.

If this trend toward body image dissatisfaction continues to grow, we ultimately may need to learn new strategies to temper our views.

We should be aware that research findings regarding body image and cosmetic surgery come out of three different generations of study, with differences that can best be reconciled if we understand that results are impacted by **a)** differences in methodologies **b)** altered societal attitudes and **c)** variations in specific thoughts and behaviors unique to each generation.

But in reviewing the research, one becomes aware that not every person benefits from cosmetic surgery. Some have inappropriate motivations. Others have expectations that are not, possibly cannot, be realized. Such is often the case for that small, but growing percentage of our population thought to be suffering from BDD (Body Dysmorphic Disorder), a condition that causes a person to be excessively distressed and preoccupied by their physical appearance. When this excessive dissatisfaction or preoccupation with a perceived defect is either imagined or highly exaggerated, that person is likely to be suffering from BDD (Body Dysmorphic Disorder).

The anorexic, a person who just can't have a thin enough body, is an extreme example of someone with an all encompassing focus on even a minimal physical defect. Depending upon the study one cites, approximately 1% - 4% of our general population is thought to suffer from BDD **25**(Crerand et al.), **26**(Phillips). Approximately ten studies have now looked into the incidences of BDD within the population of those presenting for cosmetic surgery. Collectively, the strongest studies suggest that 7% - 15% of those presenting for cosmetic surgery met BDD diagnostic criteria. **27**(Sarwer et al.)

The obsessive cosmetic surgery patient is less likely to be happy with her surgical outcome and sometimes experiences further depression afterwards because her surgical changes did not improve her feelings about her body image. This is an unfortunate experience for both patient and surgeon.

Who Gets Cosmetic Surgery Today?

People often wonder, *Is there a typical woman who goes for cosmetic surgery?* As cosmetic surgery increasingly becomes a mainstream event, 'typical' becomes harder to define. We do know that in 2005, the vast majority of the cosmetic surgery population nationwide was female (90%). Those between the ages of thirty-five to fifty represent the largest single age group for cosmetic procedures, with ages fifty-one to sixty-four next largest in size. The ethnic representation for cosmetic surgery was Caucasian 79.7%, Hispanics 9%, African American 6%, Asians 4% and other non-Caucasians 1.3%. **28**

When I asked **Denise** about the type woman who comes to her for cosmetic surgery advice, she described her clients as generally well above average in intelligence, with a keen sense of self-awareness and awareness to the responses of people who touch their lives. Although I had asked her specifically about women, Denise said she could say much the same for her male clients, whom she assures me seek cosmetic surgery at a 30% to 70 % ratio in Manhattan.

As my interviews progressed, I made many similar observations. I was impressed by how many of my interviewees' conversations reflected a love of life, a depth of intelligence and understanding – all of which drew me to them. They were generally self-actualized women who either had meaningful, productive careers or dedicated their lives to other stimulating pursuits. Those who were mothers spoke of their children as one of their most significant worldly contributions. Those who had careers spoke about the fulfillment they found in their work. They spoke of friendships, family relationships and achievements, cultural and intellectual pursuits, but they also spoke about cosmetic surgery and its impact on their self-image. Decreased self-consciousness and shyness, fewer sexual inhibitions, increased confidence and uplifted spirits were high on their lists.

Although most of these women readily admitted that they liked the feeling of looking good, they hardly seemed to fit the Webster Dictionary definition of vanity, the word so often associated with people who undergo surgery to enhance their appearance.

> *Vanity: having no real value, having an excessively high regard for one's self, for one's appearance, marked by futility or ineffectiveness, unsuccessful*

Yet it seems self evident that those who undergo such surgeries have a higher investment in their appearance, coupled with heightened dissatisfaction, than those who do not make this choice for themselves. Some individuals obviously will derive greater self-esteem from their physical appearance than others.

Most current body image research recognizes the individual's perception, (the extent to which the person is able to judge their appearance accurately) and attitudes, (an individual's thoughts, feelings and behaviors relating to their physical appearance), as critical to their body image. Sarwer et al. have identified two components to attitudes: **a)** the person's emotional experiences such as shame, disgust or anxiety as a result of their body image appraisals and **b)** body image investment, the extent to which their attentions, thoughts and actions are focused on physical appearance as a criteria for defining their sense of self. **29** There is a likely interplay of elements of both perception and attitude within most women who choose cosmetic surgery for themselves.

But because the amount of dissatisfaction with body image in our society is clearly rising, as are the statistics for Body Dysmorphic Disorder, we need to watch these trends carefully.

How Do You Know If You Have BDD?

The *Sex, Lies and Cosmetic Surgery* **CD – Part I** contains a checklist of classic symptoms of BDD. If, after referring to these criteria, you suspect that you are suffering from this disorder, I would encourage you to speak with a mental health specialist - one with a good understanding of body image dissatisfaction. You want to be absolutely certain that cosmetic surgery is the right answer for you at this time.

You should know that cosmetic surgery often leads to changes in the way people feel about themselves in addition to some more or less permanent changes to their appearance. You want to be sure that the post surgery changes you experience are positive ones and do not end up distressing you further.

Conclusions

Looking beyond the many reasons for the explosion of interest in cosmetic surgery, increased self-esteem and life optimism remain two of its widely documented benefits. There is even some evidence that the positive attitude, the renewed vitality, the vast majority of people gain from cosmetic surgery contributes to their good health and longevity.

And yet, as much as I wish for open-minded acceptance, I worry about some of the current behaviors and attitudes that I increasingly observe. For example, in their chapter on *Physical Appearance and Society*, Sarwer and Magee share anecdotal reports of young women "in select suburbs of many American cities" receiving gifts of rhinoplasty or breast augmentation surgeries to celebrate special milestones in their lives, as Sweet Sixteen birthdays or high school graduations. **30**

I laughed as I watched a TV HBO episode of *Curb Your Enthusiasm*, when a pretty blonde lifted her sweater to display her 'new boobs' and insisted that Larry David touch them to see how real they felt. The consternation on Larry's face provoked a laugh-out-loud moment for me. But I didn't find it quite so amusing when a young woman unbuttoned her blouse at my beauty salon to display her new breasts to the entire staff and surrounding clients. Some of the staff gushed: They look great. You really *needed* that surgery. It bothers me when I hear the word *need* used in conjunction with cosmetic surgery for it speaks of necessity. People *need* heart surgery, appendectomies, hernia repairs and more. But I did not *need* facial rejuvenation procedures beyond the ptosis repair, nor did the woman in the beauty salon *need* breast augmentation to remain medically healthy. Let's keep things in perspective. There are a few within the medical profession who should learn to do the same.

181

Consider this TV reality show segment, which my friend **Teresa** shared with me:

> "A woman bared her breasts – at least a size D cup if not larger - before a plastic surgeon. I thought I must have misunderstood when I heard her say that she wanted larger breasts! But I was quickly assured that my hearing was intact. It was the world that had gone berserk. The surgeon was actually nodding his head up and down and agreeing with the woman that he would recommend breast augmentation for her."

It seems to me that we as a society are caught in the midst of a whirlwind of conflicting values. There are those who, having little understanding of either body image construct or psychological underpinnings, regard cosmetic surgery as little more than an act of vanity, and are likely to react to it with feelings of embarrassment, secrecy or disdain. At the other extreme, there are some who seem to regard cosmetic surgery as the road to human perfection and focus on their physical appearance to the exclusion of other critical aspects of their being. The pendulum has swung to the right and the left. Hopefully we will find that middle ground, for any indulgence can become a vice if pursued at the expense of other virtues.

Helpful Resources

See also the following end-of-book helpful resources pertinent to information found in this chapter.

CD Part I: Self-assessment: Test Your Body Image

CD Part J: A Checklist of the Common Signs of Body Dysmorphic Disorder (BDD)

Appendix 8: Personal Profiles
(More about the people whose names appear in this chapter)

Footnotes

1. Navarra T. "Why turn our backs on plastic surgery patients?" <u>RN</u>. 49.67(2). (Feb. 1986).

2. Hill G. and Silver AG. "Psychodynamic and esthetic motivations for plastic surgery". <u>Psychosomatic Medicine</u>. 12: (1950): 345-352.

3. EdgertonMT. Jabcobson WE. and Meyer E. "Surgical-psychiatric study of patients seeking plastic (cosmetic) surgery: Ninety-eight consecutive patients with minimal deformity". <u>British Journal of Plastic Surgery</u>. 13: (1960):136-145.

4. Webb WL. Slaughter R. Meyer E. and Edgerton M. "Mechanism of psychological adjustment in patients seeking face-lift operations".<u>Psychosomatic Medicine</u>. 27(2): (1965):183-199.

5. Sarwer DB. Crerand CE. "Body image and cosmetic medical treatments". <u>Body Image: An International Journal of Research</u>, 2004;1:99-111.

6. Linni I. and Goldman IB. "Psychiatric observations concerning rhinoplasty". Psychosomatic Medicine. 11: (1949): 307-315.

7. Goin MK. Burgoyne RW. Goin JM. and Staples FR. "A prospective psychological study of 50 female face-lift patients." <u>Plastic Reconstructive Surgery</u>. 65 (1980): 436.

8. Baker JL. Jr. Kolin IS. and Bartlett ES. "Psychosexual dynamics of patients undergoing mammary augmentation." <u>Plastic Reconstructive Surgery</u>. 53. (1974): 652.

9. Goin MK. and Rees T. "A prospective study of patients' psychological reactions to rhinoplasty. " <u>Annals of Plastic Surgery</u>. 27.3. (1991): 210-215

10. Goin JM. and Goin MK. "Psychological effects of aesthetic facial surgery." <u>Advances in Psychosomatic Medicine</u>. 15. (1986).

11. Goin JM. and Goin MK. "Psychological effects of aesthetic facial surgery." <u>Advances in Psychosomatic Medicine</u>. 15. (1986): 84-108.

12.. Bank D. "A psychiatrist's view of cosmetic surgery." In. <u>Beautiful Skin: Every Woman's Guide to Looking Her Best at Any Age</u>. Adams Media Corporation. (2000): 181.

13. Maksud DP. and Anderson RC. "Psychological dimensions of aesthetic surgery: essentials for nurses." <u>Plastic Surgical Nursing</u>. 15.3. (1995): 137-144.

14. Pruzinsky T. "Psychological factors in cosmetic plastic surgery: recent developments in patient care." <u>Plastic Surgical Nursing</u>. 13.2.: 64-70.

15. Spira M. and Scheck A. "Changing beauty ideals impact cosmetic surgery." <u>Cosmetic Surgery Times.</u> 4.4 (May 2001): 14.

16. Sarwer DB. and Magee L. "Physical appearance and society". In. <u>Psychological Aspects of Reconstructive and Cosmetic Plastic Surgery: Clinical, Empirical and Ethical Perspectives</u>. Lippincott, Williams and Wilkens (Sept. 2005): 31.

17. Profile of the Nation's Health Book. Department of Health and Human Services, The Centers for Disease Control (CDC) and Prevention Fact Book and The National Center for Health Statistics – Fast Stats – Life Expectancy.

18. Central Intelligence Agency (CIA). World Fact Book.2005

19. http//www.census.gov/statab/www/pop.html

20. Monteath S. and McCabe M. "The influence of societal factors on female body image." <u>The Journal of Social Psychology</u>. 137 (Dec.1997): 708-27.

21. Fredrickson B. and Robert T. "Objectification theory – toward understanding women's lived experiences and mental health risks." <u>Psychology of Women Quarterly.</u> 21 (1997): 173-206.

22. Sarwer DB. and Magee L. "Physical appearance and society". In. **Psychological Aspects of Reconstructive and Cosmetic Plastic Surgery: Clinical, Empirical and Ethical Perspectives**. Lippincott, Williams and Wilkens (Sept. 2005): 23-36.

23. Sarwer DB. et al. eds. **Psychological Aspects of Reconstructive and Cosmetic Plastic Surgery: Clinical, Empirical and Ethical Perspectives**, Lippincott. Williams and Wilkens (Sept. 2005): 236.

24. Fetto J. "Image is everything." **American Demographics**. 25.2 (March 2003): 10-11.

25. Crerand CE. Cash TF. and Whitaker LA. "Cosmetic surgery of the face." In. **Psychological Aspects of Reconstructive and Cosmetic Plastic Surgery: Clinical, Empirical and Ethical Perspectives**. Lippincott, Williams and Wilkens (Sept. 2005): 242.

26. Phillips K. **The Broken Mirror: Understanding and Treating Body Dysmorphic Disorder**. NewYork: Oxford University Press. (1996).

27. Sarwer DB. Wadden T. Pertschuk M. Whitaker I. "The psychology of cosmetic surgery: a review and reconceptualization" **Clinical Psychol Rev** (1998): 1-22.

28. American Society of Aesthetic Plastic Surgery (ASAPS). 2005 statistics. http://www.surgery.org/press/statistics.asp

29. Cash TF. "Psychology of physical appearance" In. **Psychological Aspects of Reconstructive and Cosmetic Plastic Surgery: Clinical, Empirical and Ethical Perspectives**. Lippincott, Williams and Wilkens (Sept. 2005): 39.

30. Sarwer DB. and Magee L. "Physical appearance and society". In. **Psychological Aspects of Reconstructive and Cosmetic Plastic Surgery: Clinical, Empirical and Ethical Perspectives**, Lippincott. Williams and Wilkens (Sept. 2005): 31.

The Short Story:

Two different perspectives of our world of the not-too-distant future

"Satire: A literary work holding up human vices or follies to ridicule or scorn."

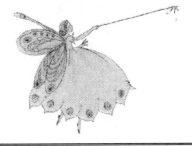

Please take this trip with me into two very different worlds of the twilight zone. Decide for yourself where cosmetic surgery fits into your thinking. Do you want to swim with the tide, float on your back or fight the current?

Step Right

It's the year 2025. Please forego reality for a moment to enter this time and place where each person's physical attributes are judged purely by perceived accomplishment, not by any of our current standards of beauty. How divine! Drooping eyelids are now a subject of admiration. Is it any wonder? The woman with eyes nearly hidden beneath mounds of extra flesh must have absorbed a vast assortment of lifetime images. All at once you envision her as an accomplished artist and her inner beauty nearly explodes in your mind. As you turn slightly clockwise, you are immediately drawn to the man with significant love handles. In your fantasies you envision him as a gourmand who has created and savored many of the world's epicurean delights. His perceived talents are so seductive! You are suddenly distracted once again – this time by the sight of a woman standing aside with protruding abdomen and sagging breasts. Your heart skips a beat. How alluring she appears! After all, aren't women placed on earth to procreate and suckle babies? This woman must have done more than her share.

Of course, these are only first impressions. You may change your mind a bit as you get to know these people better. But in this world, these three people will receive preferential treatment in many spheres of life, based purely on this society's perception of their life experiences and accomplishments. One's unique physical attributes are seen as nothing more than an extension of who they are by way of what they have accomplished.

An occasional societal member wanders astray, actually seeks ways to modify her appearance, camouflage the very essence of who she is. This pathology is treated with intense Behavior Modification Therapy as well as anti-depressant medications.

Does this sound like science fiction? If this fantasy world is not to your liking, please follow me into the next world of the *twilight zone.*

Step Left

We are still in the year 2025. Please come right in. You are about to enter a society highly focused on aesthetics. While still in your teens, your mother will schedule your first appointment with your plastic surgeon. At this time you will be given a comprehensive, three-dimensional computerized body mapping in a devise similar in appearance to the MRI equipment of today. A second machine will record the exact contours of your face, the texture and tautness of your skin. Your surgeon will modify the appearance of your eyes, your chin, your nose, your breasts . . . , right on the computer screen, to show you how closely he can surgically alter your features to conform to current standards of beauty. He will use his artistry and experience to help guide you toward selections suited to your face, your body type and your vision.

Different sizes, shapes and contours of noses await your inspection in the nose cabinet, whereas a full array of breasts of various sizes, degrees of fullness and cleavage depths can be found behind the doors of the breast cabinet. The final choice rests with you.

If you are among the chosen few of exceptional post surgical beauty, your doctor will invite you to participate in the regional beauty pageant of the surgically enhanced. Winners of these regional competitions move up to the statewide level and finally to that broadly televised, eagerly awaited national competition. Victors of this final competition become the socially elite. There is no more coveted prize to be earned by a woman or her plastic surgeon.

Let's stop and reflect for a moment on these two scenarios, each a vast exaggeration of fact, each nonetheless slightly reflective of current views both left and right of center.

Lucille sent the following words as her sole written response to my cosmetic surgery questionnaire:

> "After having my own appearance ruined by plastic surgery, I have come to the conclusion that doctors who operate on people with normal anatomy for monetary gain are not practicing MEDICINE at all. I now believe it is unethical for doctors to place people in harms way with unnecessary surgery. Plastic

surgeons should be confined to using their skills on deformities from disease, congenital defects and trauma and refuse to operate on patients with NORMAL anatomy."

Her words clearly reflect a right of center viewpoint. I was unsuccessful in my attempts to contact **Lucille** through the e-mail address she had provided. Had I achieved contact, I would have asked for the name of her surgeon to check out his credentials. I also would have inquired about her motivations and outcome expectations. Without that information, I am left with pure conjecture. Perhaps she made a poor choice when selecting the physician to perform her surgery. Perhaps she had unrealistic expectations or experienced an unfortunate complication. But I will never know for sure.

Although **Abby's** words were not nearly so harsh, they still veer slightly right of center:

"If people would only focus more on developing their inner selves, their personalities, their values, their concern for others, they would begin to focus less on their appearance. I think that would be helpful to the individual and to society as a whole."

In some ways I agree with **Abby.** It would be pure utopia to be living in that kinder, gentler world she describes, the one **Harriet Spitzer** and **Linda Novick** spoke about in Chapter 8, *What Deters Us.*

Next we have **Fran Orgovan,** the esthetician you met in several previous chapters, whose artistic eye leads her to envision the potential for beauty in each human form. Her favorite hobby of painting nudes has helped shape her somewhat left of center perspective about cosmetic surgery. "When I watch a plastic surgeon during surgery, I think of the patient's face or body as the artist's canvas and the surgeon as the artist at work. To me cosmetic surgery is a series of skilled techniques designed to enhance the beauty of the human form."

Grace, the fifty year old cosmetic saleswoman from Staten Island, NY shared a similar, but slightly more centered philosophy:

> "I thought to myself that fashions come and go. Clothing styles quickly become outdated. But I am going to wear my face all day every day for the rest of my life, so I might as well enjoy my face."

In Chapter 11, *Changing Attitudes – From Freud too the 21st Century,* you read about many of the reasons why there has been a gradual shift in perspective – an attitude that increasingly embraces the right for individuals to alter their appearance. More and more, cosmetic surgery is being regarded as a reasonable, even desirable option for people who want to improve the way they look. Malcolm Paul, MD, President of the California Society of Plastic Surgeons (2005-2006) and Past President of the American Society for Aesthetic Plastic Surgery, explains it this way:

> *People today generally are not ashamed to admit that they care about their appearance, and they enjoy having the freedom to make choices about how they want to look.*

That beautiful hair stylist, **Val**, clearly agrees.

> "You know and I know that it is inevitable – God willing, we are all going to grow old. I feel in the process, if it makes you feel better to enhance the way you look, why not? Some people are just as happy to grow old naturally. Good for them! Unfortunately, or fortunately, at this point in my life, I am not one of them."

National Trends

Each year increasing numbers of people are having cosmetic procedures and treatments. According to the latest statistics compiled by the ASAPS, based on a survey sent to nearly eight thousand physicians nationwide, the number of cosmetic procedures performed in the United States from 1997-2005 has increased by 444%. Nearly 11.5 million cosmetic *surgical and non-surgical* procedures were performed in the year 2005, with nearly 10.5 million of them performed on women.

> "More and more people are having procedures and treatments done at an earlier age. As these procedures become less invasive and time consuming than in past years, and as we as a society are more conscious about our health and appearance, the acceptance and popularity of 'getting something done' is growing. The easier and quicker 'lunch time' procedures, such as Botox, microdermabrasion, and collagen fit well into today's busy lifestyle." 1

The chart below provides a quick overview of the surgical and non-surgical procedures that headed the U.S. popularity hit parade in the year 2005. 2

Surgical Procedures	Number Performed on females	% Change Since 1997
Liposuction	455,489	+171%
Breast augmentation	364,610	+260%
Eyelid surgery	231,467	+46%
Rhinoplasty (nose)	200,924	+67%
Facelifts	150,401	+55%
Tummy Tuck	169,314	+400%
Breast reduction	160,531	+235%

Non-Surgical Procedure	Number Performed	% Change Since 2003
Botox injections	3,294,782	+4,893%
Laser hair removal	1,566,909	NA
Chemical Peels	566,172	+18%
Microdermabrasion	1,023,931	NA
Hyaluronic Acid (Hylaform, Restylane)	1,194,222	NA

You can see from these statistics that there is an upward trend in all cosmetic *surgical* procedures, with liposuction, breast augmentation and eyelid repairs the most frequently performed surgical procedures. In the *non-surgical* arena, Botox, laser hair removal and Hylaform/Restylane top the list.

Have We Gone Too Far?

Jack M. Gorman, M.D., Professor of Psychiatry at Columbia University, expresses his thoughts on this subject.

> "Many of us try to alter our appearance by dieting and exercise. These are widely considered positive and healthy actions, yet they still represent efforts to alter the natural state of our physical existence. As long as expectations are realistic, cosmetic surgery seems to me to be part and parcel of the same concept – the important role in our lives of looking (and feeling) good." **3**

To a large extent, I agree. I want us to continue to endorse an accepting attitude toward altering our appearance by surgical or non-surgical means. I would feel repressed if our current attitudes were undermined to the point where people once again were intimidated into accepting that *don't tamper with what nature provides* philosophy. There is no reason for quiet acceptance or unhealthy resignation just to adhere to societal dictates.

But I think we need to be realistic and recognize that cosmetic procedures are not a panacea for all of life's ills. We also should not lose sight of the fact that cosmetic surgery is still surgery and that good health should remain our first consideration.

Gail, the professional singer who prefers quiet dinners and intimate fireside conversations, tempers her enthusiasm for cosmetic surgery with her belief that if you have health problems that could compromise a successful outcome, you shouldn't risk it.

> "After all, this is elective surgery and there are many other joys one can experience in life besides appearance enhancements. But if you are in good health and think it is something that would give you pleasure, why not? It's a great gift to give yourself."

Despite words of caution, the media pendulum continues to swing left of center: reality television shows of women undergoing radical, multiple surgical procedures, beauty pageants with surgically altered contestants competing against one another; fashion shows of post surgery patients modeling their enhanced appearances before appreciative, live audiences and an all too eager press ready to fulfill career driven desires for publicity. Some women have become so transfixed by the hype that they return year after year for just one more psychic-cosmetic fix.

Can't we maintain some semblance of balance? Why does that non-celebrity status person, one with no professional need for physical perfection, feel a need to refine normal features into perfect ones, when those surgeries will have minimal to no effect on overall facial appearance? For example, does a nose that isn't chiseled to perfection, which has a regular shape, average length, no bumps and is only slightly imperfect, really call out for cosmetic surgery? My mom used to preach: "Everything in moderation." I hope we do indeed heed those words and not go too far.

Teresa, the psychiatric social worker you met in Chapter 11, *Changing Attitudes From Freud to the 21st Century,* sent me the following note several days after enjoying dinner together:

> ". . . Please let me clear up one misconception I inadvertently may have conveyed to you. I'm not against cosmetic surgery per se – not at all. What I meant is, I think it gets out of bounds when individuals get obsessed with it to the point that they feel they need to "fix" almost every facial or body part they have in an endless quest to look like models or movie stars. I do wish those individuals would work on their emotional selves more, as there is something wrong when a person needs to do that – a decided lack of self-esteem and self-love within themselves. . . . But when someone is unhappy with how they look or wants a pick-up or enhancement, that's fine - why not? I just think that extremes in anything are not desirable."

Her words once again speak to that *everything in moderation* philosophy.

Only you can answer the question: "Where does cosmetic surgery fit into my life?" For some, the answer will be "It doesn't." Others will regard it as a reasonable, viable option of equal legitimacy.

Helpful Resources

See also the following end-of-book helpful resources
pertinent to information found in this chapter.

☼   **Appendix 8: Personal Profiles**
     (More about the people whose
     names appear in this chapter)

Footnotes

1. Bank D. Beautiful Skin: Every Woman's Guide to Looking Her Best at Any Age. Adams Media Corporation. (2000): 245-246.

2. All cited statistics have been compiled by the American Society for Aesthetic Plastic Surgery (ASAPS).

3. Gorman J "A psychiatrist's view of cosmetic surgery." In. Bank D. Beautiful Skin: Every Woman's Guide to Looking Her Best at Any Age. Adams Media Corporation. (2000): 181.

Chapter 13: Brain Sex, Women and Cosmetic Surgery

The Short Story:

Conjecture - Is There a Relationship Between the Structure of the Female Brain, Sexuality and Cosmetic Surgery?

"Conjecture: Inferences made from Presumptive Evidence"

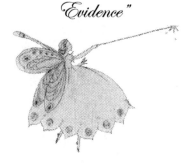

Since I opened this book with a joke, it now seems fitting that as I near its conclusion, I begin similarly. I suspect this joke that will resonate with men and women alike.

> A man is strolling along the beaches of California when he hears turbulence up above, looks skyward and sees God before him. "You have been such a virtuous man all your life, that I want to reward you," says God. "I will grant you any one wish that your heart desires." The man thinks for awhile and then responds, "Oh, God, if only you could build a bridge from here to Hawaii. How I would love to take long hikes across the Pacific Ocean to reach the Hawaiian shores."

199

God is very quiet for a moment and then responds,

> "Do you realize what a difficult task you are asking of me? Think of the tons of steel this would require. And those cement pilings – they would have to be plunged so deeply into the ocean to secure such a bridge. Perhaps you can think of another wish that won't be so difficult for me to fulfill."

The man agrees that he will think some more.

A week goes by and once again God makes his presence known. "Have you thought of another wish that I might grant you?" asks God.

> "Yes, God, I have", says the man. "If only you could help me understand my wife better. Sometimes she is so loving, but at other times, for no apparent reason, she turns away from me if I try to touch her or simply bursts into tears. When she's in such a state, lovemaking becomes impossible. Life would be nearly perfect if I could only change this situation. Please, God, can you help me understand her better?"

God pauses, deep in thought before he finally responds, "Was it two lanes or four that you wanted on that bridge to Hawaii?"

The point to this joke is rather clear, for simple observation of human behavior tells us that men and women typically function differently in the emotional and sexual domains. But before I speak in terms of gender specific differences, I need to begin with a disclaimer.

> *Generalizations are never hard and fast rules. Some competing evidence normally can be found to refute almost any statement, no matter how much supporting data exists for its validity.*

For example, we can state that men are usually taller than women. Statistically this is a fact as on average, men are 7% taller than women. But exceptions certainly exist. Some women are obviously going to be taller than some men. The same will be true of my next statements about the differences in the way male and female brains typically function, because there are men and women whose brains do not function as the *typical* male/female patterns I am about to describe. So I urge you to keep in mind that the following information is factual yet non-definite. Although these next expressed generalizations are stated in terms of the *average* male and *average* female, know that as with all generalizations, exceptions will occur.

John Gray raised our consciousness about many of these male/female differences in his series of Mars and Venus books, beginning with Men Are From Mars, Women Are From Venus. He spoke about actual biochemical differences in our brains that affect our sexual functioning. [1] For example, he explained that the typical male is stimulated to produce greater supplies of the brain hormone, dopamine, at the beginning of a new relationship. He becomes attentive, with increased eye contact and produces plenty of testosterone. Gray further explains that when the newness of a relationship levels off, so does the body's production of dopamine, often encouraging this same man to seek out exciting new situations or take further risks to try to recapture his previous high.

He contrasts this scenario with that of the woman, who is typically controlled by her serotonin levels. According to Gray, this brain neurotransmitter that gives a woman feelings of contentment, relaxation and optimism, is primarily stimulated by the quality of her relationships. Low levels of serotonin inhibit a woman's ability to nurture, understand and trust, the very elements which stimulate female sexuality.

"Low serotonin levels also dramatically affect romantic relationships. . . . Most qualities and characteristics that men love about women are enriched with normal serotonin levels." **2**

As I mentally sorted through this information, three questions came to mind: **a)** What causes male and female brains to function differently? **b)** Can these gender specific differences explain why women undergo the vast majority of cosmetic surgeries? **c)** How much do all of these gender specific factors - brain structures, brain function and incidences of cosmetic surgery - relate to female sexuality? Let's look at these questions one at a time.

What Causes Typical Differences in Male and Female Brain Functions?

"Each mammal, from mole to man, is shaped by sex hormones in the womb." **3**

In 1991, Anne Moir and David Jessel published a compilation of brain research that they had gathered from many quarters of the world. Their book, <u>Brain Sex - The Real Difference Between Men and Women</u>, reported on a large number of studies into the *structural* differences between male and female brains. The evidence from these diverse studies was both dramatic and conclusive, yet those who initiated these studies were so geographically scattered that few knew of the existence of other studies with similar outcomes. **4**

What I learned from these studies is that male and female brains typically *function* differently because they are *structured* differently. Here are the facts as explained by Moir and Jessel:

The brains of humans begin to take shape about 6-8 weeks after conception. In the normal XY blueprint, *if all goes as planned*, embryonic boys develop special cells that produce male hormones, mainly testosterone, and male genitals. At that critical time in their development, boy embryos are exposed to huge surges of male hormones – actually four times the amount they receive throughout infancy and boyhood. They do not experience such a surge again until adolescence. *It is that surge of testosterone in the developing male fetus that alters the actual structure of the baby boy's brain.*

In the normal XX blueprint, *if all goes as planned*, no master switch is turned on. The fetus continues to grow and develop without dramatic change. The female embryo, the XX, receives only small amounts of testosterone. This female brain seems to be the default pattern, the one that develops unless hormones intervene to alter its structure. In other words, this female brain pattern is altered only when the fetus receives large doses of testosterone at its crucial time of development.

In the past, behavioral differences between the sexes were often dismissed as social conditioning (e.g. differential treatment, differential expectations and differential messages society bestowed on our sons and daughters). Today there is too much science, too much biological evidence, for this sociological argument to prevail. Studies of groups of people with anomalies to their sexual development as a result of specific hormone deficiencies, described in the addendum at the end of this chapter, provide convincing evidence of biology over environment.

Science continues to document structural and functional differences in the male and female brain. One well documented difference confirms the fact that the left and right sides of a woman's brain are more integrated. In other words, both the left and right hemispheres of her brain are typically involved in verbal, visual and emotional responses. The two sides of the man's brain are more specialized, with his left side almost exclusively in control of verbal abilities. His right side controls visual responses and abstract problem solving. These sex linked differences in brain structure have been repeatedly documented through measurements of electrical brain activity while men and women executed specific tasks. I was intrigued to discover that the amount of testosterone the fetus receives during embryonic development has a decided impact not just on the brain's structure, but on its actual functioning as well.

The structure of our brain impacts on how we respond to emotions. Men's emotional responses are specific to the right hemisphere. Women's are more diffuse, centered within both the right and left hemispheres. Furthermore, the corpus callosum, the bundle of fibers that serves as the message exchange center between our left and right hemispheres, is thicker and more bulbous in women. This structure enables the two sides of the female brain to exchange more information. These organic, structural differences add credence to the results of other studies that conclude that women in general are better at sensory intake and consequently more readily able to recognize the emotional nuances of voice, gesture, facial expressions, body language, etc.

Both sides of the typical female brain have the capacity for emotional response. *Because more emotional information is exchanged between the two sides of the woman's brain and what she feels is transmitted and integrated within her verbal left front hemisphere, she generally feels and expresses her emotions more readily.*

Men typically keep their emotions on the right side of their brains, separate from the left hemisphere speech centers. **5** Furthermore, since his two hemispheres are connected by a narrower corpus callosum with fewer neural fibers, the flow of information between one side of his brain and the other is more restricted. *It isn't simply that in general men have* *greater difficulty expressing emotions. They actually receive less emotional intake.*

The male and female brains not only *feel* emotions differently, they also *see* things differently. Structurally, women have more receptor rods and cones in their retina, which enables them to receive a wider arc of visual input and provides them with greater peripheral vision. Generally, whereas the female brain receives a wider arc of sensory information enabling women to take in the bigger picture, men tend to see things in a narrow field, with greater concentration and depth.

Simon Baron Cohen, a professor of psychology and psychiatry at the University of Cambridge, has added to our understanding of male and female brain differences with his thesis that *the typical male brain is predominantly hard-wired for understanding and building systems, whereas the typical female brain is predominantly hard-wired for empathy.* **6** He draws on clinical case studies and scientific research to explain why men are better at analyzing and building abstract systems and woman are better at empathizing and communicating. Baron Cohen further defines these differences of the male 'systematic' brain and the female 'empathetic' brain as more biological than cultural.

Other studies specifying similar sex linked differences conclude that females on average are better at interpreting body language, verbal tone and facial expression (Hall) **7** and that females also are better at interpreting the subtle mental states of others by regarding the eye region of their faces (Baron-Cohen et. al.) **8** Further interesting findings are emerging from a series of ongoing studies at the University of Cambridge, where mothers undergoing amniocentesis granted researchers permission to analyze their fetal fluid and later take part in a study designed to test for correlations between fetal testosterone levels and subsequent language development, social relationships, interests and more. Findings from these studies suggest that lower levels of fetal testosterone (generally found in the female fetus) correlate positively with newborn babies' greater interest in human faces, as opposed to mechanical mobiles. Higher fetal testosterone levels, (generally found in the male fetus), correlate positively with less eye contact at 12 months of age and lower empathy quotient scores at 6-9 years of age. **9**

Do Gender Specific Brain Differences Relate to Women's Attraction to Cosmetic Surgery?

Since there is rather conclusive scientific evidence that male and female brains are *structured* differently and to that degree also *function* differently, it makes perfect sense to me that:

• The person whose brain is more finely tuned to receive nuances of meaning from subtle social interactions (e.g. body language, facial expressions, subtle verbal messages, voice tone, media hype) is going to be more tuned to how others respond to her. Experiences the male brain simply does not absorb are more likely to penetrate that female brain. (Remember, generally the female brain receives a freer flow of emotional data and a wider arc of sensory information.) I suspect that men are more oblivious to the casual comment, facial expression, mirror image or photograph that often serves as a female impetus for cosmetic change. As we saw in Chapter 11, *Changing Attitudes From Freud to the 21st Century*, none of this is lost on the media, which expends the vast portion of its resources to capitalize on this female consciousness about appearance and to heighten her beauty standards and self-expectations for beauty.

• The person whose brain places a higher priority on personal relationships has a stronger desire to reach out to others and have those gestures of acceptance reciprocated, even in casual interactions. Not only does the female brain more readily pick up on those subtleties, but women seem to have a stronger emotional response to them.

• The person whose brain is more emotionally responsive has more of a *need* for nurturance on many levels, including a greater need for gestures of acceptance in interpersonal relationships and the nurturance that comes back to her from a more positive physical self-image. Men's brains generally have a lesser need for all types of nurturance, including that garnered from their physical being. Generally studies conclude that men are more likely to seek empowerment through achievement, dominance and accomplishment and that these are the very traits that attract women to them. Nurturance from others and appearance related boosts to self-esteem are much further down on the male priority list.

Women's greater awareness of social nuances and their stronger need for emotional nurturance seem like two logical explanations for statistics showing that the vast majority of all cosmetic surgeries are performed on women. **10**

Do Gender Specific Brain Differences Impact Sexuality After Cosmetic Surgery?

To establish scientific fact, one normally begins with a premise to explain a specific phenomenon, and then subjects that tentative explanation to scientific investigation. Armed with the information about sex linked brain differences, I began to form a tentative theory of my own:
Perhaps the emotional high many women experience after cosmetic surgery stimulates increased serotonin production.

I posed the following question to several endocrinologists:
Can women's strong positive emotions result in increased production of serotonin?

None of them had ever heard of such a theory, therefore what I am left with is pure conjecture based on presumptive evidence, and should not be construed as scientific fact. But I wonder if it is possible that women - those generally more tuned to nuances of meaning from subtle social interactions, ordinarily placing a higher priority on both personal relationships and nurturance – could be more sexually impacted by positive post surgery emotions, be they internally or externally aroused?

Results of good cosmetic surgery add to most women's positive thoughts and feelings in two ways: Women are aroused internally by that feel good feeling their improved appearance brings their way. They also are aroused externally by the positive feedback they get from others. Could women also experience a boost to their serotonin levels, that hormonal component to female sexuality, as a result of their post surgery emotional highs?
I don't know the answer to this question; but I suspect that the sexual impact for women is typically stronger than that experienced by men, who are stimulating to arousal quite differently.

> "Voyeuristic porn and its capacity to stun the brain might adjust male capability in bed but it does not much influence that of the female. A woman's arousal is extremely person and environment specific." 11

So far research primarily has centered on several specific aspects of sex linked functional differences as spatial abilities, play interests and verbal skills. Although research has touched on emotional differences as well, more concentrated work in this area is needed before science can either confirm or negate my conjectures about gender specific brain differences and their impact on sexuality after cosmetic surgery.

But who knows? Perhaps that virtuous man who asked God to build him a bridge to Hawaii, would have been better served by asking God to reveal some of these yet untapped aspects of gender specific brain differences.

Addendum: Studies - When Things Go Wrong in Brain Development

Many of the male and female brain studies have been performed on rats. The results of these studies and the observations they engender are interesting, but one questions how closely they apply to the far more complex human brain. Scientific studies on human brains obviously are harder to conduct. Several of particular relevancy have looked at groups of people hit with unusual concentrations of sex hormones during brain development.

CAH (congenital adrenal hyperplasia) is a condition caused by a genetic defect of the adrenal gland, resulting in female fetus exposure to high levels of masculinizing steroid hormones. As a result, at birth their female genitals take on the size and shape of male organs. This male appearance of their female genitals is normally surgically corrected at birth and the girls are given hormone therapy to curtail any further testosterone effects. These CAH babies prove to be female as they have all the appropriate female internal organs of ovaries, fallopian tubes and a uterus. The CAH girl can live a normal female life. With the assistance of hormone therapy, she can go through puberty on schedule and even become pregnant and give birth to children.

> "Researchers who studied female victims of CAH discovered that despite the earliest of interventions, these girls exhibited play habits similar to those of boys. They preferred rough, energetic games and outdoor play." **12**

As they matured, CAH females scored significantly higher in tests of spatial abilities, a proven strength of the typical male brain, than did their non CAH relatives in the study.

Berenbaum, a psychologist at the Chicago Medical School, studied the play patterns of groups of children between the ages of three and eight, including two dozen CAH girls. When Berenbaum analyzed the videotaped sessions of these children's unsupervised free play, she determined that the CAH girls acted similarly to boys in their selection of toys and their manner of play. For example, they played with boys' toys more than twice as frequently as those of girls, the exact proportion of choice measured for the videotaped boys in the study. Here was an ideal group to study. Raised from birth as girls, yet exposed to exceptionally high doses of male hormones in the womb, Berenbaum theorized that since these CAH girls would have been socialized as girls, differences in their play preferences would be due to the effects of hormones at a critical point in brain development, rather than due to the effects of socialization.

> "After testing and rejecting other possible explanations for their behavior, Berenbaum has concluded that these girls' preference for trucks and Lincoln logs over dolls and toy blenders must have been caused by something male hormones did to their developing brains." 13

Berenbaum wanted to test her theories further. She knew that males rather consistently outscored females on tests of spatial orientation, including mental rotations. Although her study originated in Minnesota, she soon moved to Chicago where she further pursued her research at Chicago Medical School. Her colleague, Susan Resnick, continued Berenbaum's work at the University of Minnesota, where it had originated. Neither woman found differences in intelligence between the CAH and non CAH groups. But at both sites the CAH females scored significantly higher on tests of spatial abilities than their non CAH female relatives, with scores much closer to the males in these studies.

> "How could a shot of testosterone before birth help a person perform better on tests of spatial reasoning twelve or fifteen years later? One way is that hormones in the womb might modify the wiring of the brain, improving some skills and perhaps worsening others." **14**

The researchers continued their study by administering a questionnaire about individuals' preferred activities during childhood. They found that on average the CAH females as well as the males were less interested in verbal skills such as word games, creating stories, conversing with adults, etc. and instead seemed to prefer building models and moving objects around.

In CAH girls, and presumably in males as well, testosterone in the womb masculinizes several mental and psychological traits – play activities, spatial abilities and even choice of toys. **15**

In marked contrast to the CAH woman, whose exposure to testosterone has been excessive, lies the XY woman, who has received zero testosterone exposure. The XY woman is a genetically male person who develops more or less as a woman, minus ovaries and a uterus. These two diverse groups have served as excellent study counterpoints to one another. **16**

In 1979, a researcher from Cornell University Medical College, Julianne Imperato-McGinley, investigated the victims of two feminizing syndromes that affect genetic males. One such anomaly group was the XY women discussed in the previous paragraph, who are genetically male, but produce no male hormones and develop as women. Since XY women look completely female at birth, they are raised and socialized as girls. Thus if socialization were a determinant of differences in test scores between males and females, the XY women should score like other women, with lower spatial ability scores than men. Their spatial ability scores were indeed lower, surprisingly even lower than their 'normal' XX female relatives. Imperato-McGinley gives the following explanation:

> "Male hormones in the womb do improve a person's spatial ability, and even a small amount has an effect. Although normal females are not exposed to nearly as much male hormone during development as ('normal') males, they still do get a low dose of hormones, and that seems to be enough to give them an advantage over those who, in practical terms, get absolutely no male hormones at all." 17

The second studied victims of a feminizing syndrome that affects genetic males was a group of interrelated males living in isolated areas of the Caribbean, Dominican Republic and New Guinea, who suffered from a rare condition whereby they appeared female at birth but developed testes and a penis at puberty. These individuals were exposed to normal levels of testosterone in utero, but denied exposure to other needed male hormones. As a result, their male sex organs did not emerge until adolescence with that adolescent surge of testosterone.

At the clinic where Imperato-McGinley worked, a joke circulated amongst her colleagues, who claimed that there was no need to give a chromosome test to separate the XY women from those in the group of interrelated Caribbean males. They claimed you could simply give them a jigsaw puzzle to complete. The second group, who suffered from that rare condition whereby they appeared female at birth but developed testes and a penis at puberty, seemed to really enjoy solving those jigsaw puzzles, attacked two thousand piece puzzles with gusto and appeared to do at least as well on them as other males. Such was not the case with the XY women who were genetically male, but produced no male hormones. They exhibited difficulty piecing together even a one hundred piece puzzle and complained that doing so gave them a headache. Whereas the first victim group lacked only the hormone dihydrotestoterone, the XY women produced no male hormones at all. This information narrows the hormone field responsible for increased capacity for working jigsaw puzzles and doing mental rotations to testosterone.

One further genetic/hormonal abnormality that sheds light on brain functioning comes to us from the Turner Women. These women, whose genetic make-up is XO, are missing one of two XX female sex chromosomes. The Turner Women Society of the United States has described Turner Syndrome (TS) as "a chromosomal disorder found in females, caused by complete or partial absence of or by structural defects to the second sex chromosome, occuring in approximately 1 in 2,000 live female births. As a result of TS women's genetic composition, their gonads fail to develop into ovaries and their bodies get very minimal amounts of sex hormones. The normal female fetus produces tiny amounts of testosterone, but since the Turner Woman has no ovaries, no male hormone reaches the developing brain of the TS fetus. Consequently these women exhibit exaggeratedly female behaviors. As could be predicted,

Turner Women normally do as well on tests of verbal skills as XX women, but perform especially poorly on tests of spatial skills.

"Their problems in getting lost are legendary amongst sex researchers. Once again: minimal male hormones, minimum spatial ability." **18**

Footnotes:

1. Gray J. The Mars and Venus Diet and Exercise Solution. St. Martin's Press. (2003): 63.

2. Gray J. The Mars and Venus Diet and Exercise Solution. St. Martin's Press. (2003): 63.

3. Poole R. Eve's Rib, The Biological Roots of Sex Differences. Crown Publishers. Inc. (1994): 4.

4. Moir A. and Jessel D. Brain Sex The Real Difference Between Men and Women. First Carol Publishing Group. (1991): 24.

5. Witleson SF. "An exchange on gender." New York Review. 24 (Oct. 1985): 53-55.

6. Baron-Cohen S. The Essential Difference: The Truth About the Male and Female Brain. Perseus Books Group. (2003).

7. Hall. J. "Gender effects in decoding non-verbal cues". Psychological Bulletin. 85.(1978): 845-858.

8. Knickmeyer R. Baron-Cohen S. Raggatt P. and Taylor K. "Foetal testosterone, social relationships, and restricted interests in children" Journal of Child Psychology and Psychiatry. 46:2 (2005): 198-210.

9. Lutchmaya S. Baron-Cohen S. and Raggan P. "Foetal Testosterone and eye contact in 12-month-old human infants" Infant Behavior and Development 25 (2002): 327-335.

10. American Society for Aesthetic Plastic Surgery (ASAPS) Statistics. 2005.

11. Cook M. "Sex is back on the brain." http://www.news.scotsman.com/health.cfm?id=142032005

12. Poole R. Eve's Rib. The Biological Roots of Sex Differences. Crown Publishers. Inc. (1994): 86.

13. Berenbaum.S. and Hines R. "Early Androgens are related to childhood sex typed toy preferences". Psychological Science. 3.3 (1992): 203-206.

14. Poole R. Eve's Rib. The Biological Roots of Sex Differences. Crown Publishers. Inc. (1994): 88.

15. Poole R. Eve's Rib. The Biological Roots of Sex Differences. Crown Publishers. Inc. (1994): 91.

16. Imperato-McGinley J. Peterson R. Gautier T. and Sturla E. "Androgens and the evolution of male-gender identity among male pseudohermaphrodites with 5 $c\alpha$ – reductase deficiency". The New England Journal of Medicine.300:22 (1979): 1233-1237.

17. Imperato-McGinley J. Pichardo M. Gauter T. Voyer D. and Bryden P. "Cognitive abilities in androgen-insensitive subjects: comparison with control males and females with the same kindred". Cliinical Endocrinology.34 (1991): 341-347.

18. Poole R. Eve's Rib, The Biological Roots of Sex Differences. Crown Publishers. Inc. (1994): 101-102.

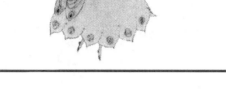
My Journey – A Circuitous Route

I was seated in the waiting room of the ophthalmic surgeon's office when I spotted a rack of brochures. I picked up one on laser resurfacing and was impressed by the pictured results. As long as I needed eyelid repair surgery, why not a little simultaneous cosmetic enhancement, I mused. Just a blip of a thought at the moment, but following my examination I took a deep breath, looked the surgeon in the eye and asked this most difficult question:

> "Dr. R . . . , I want you to look at my face and be honest with me", I began. "You have had experience with this. If I had laser resurfacing, do you think it would make a big, moderate or only slight difference in my overall appearance?"

Much to his credit, he answered me with equal honesty.

> "Picture a wrinkled tablecloth. You can iron it and take away its surface wrinkles. But if the underlying table is not smooth, the tablecloth still won't lie flat. As we age, the underlying muscles (the table) weaken. That's a good part of what makes the skin wrinkle and sag. Between ages twenty and thirty, we see very slight changes. But between ages sixty and seventy those changes become dramatic. I don't think laser resurfacing is going to give you the resolution you are looking for. And I don't want you to be disappointed later on. Why not just do your eyes? That will give you a nice, refreshed look."

"What about this area?", I asked, pointing to my lower face and neck. "Is there anything you can do to improve that?"

> "What you're really talking about here is a facelift. I don't do facelifts, but I'd be glad to recommend someone if that's what you want. We often team up together. I do the eyes, he does the rest."

The word *facelift* hit with the shock of a full bucket of ice water. Slowly I allowed this thought to penetrate. I had reached that age where decided changes in my appearance actually were starting to take place. Maybe this was what I wanted. Maybe this was what I should do.

The bait had been set. A slow even tug was reeling me in. I went for a consultation with Dr. S..., the recommended plastic surgeon, whose office was based in a rather upscale Long Island community. His waiting room and inner office wall hangings could have challenged the taste of many decorator magazines. Objects of art were strategically placed on tables within these rooms. Somehow, although I admired his taste, the formality of his office made me a bit uncomfortable. When I entered his examining room, he told me that if I had cosmetic surgery, I would always look ten years younger than all my friends. That wasn't my motivation and I was immediately turned off by his brand of salesmanship. The actual consultation was routine. He recommended a full facelift, leaving the eye work to the ophthalmic surgeon who had recommended him, explaining that they would work together as a team. I didn't like the idea of two separate surgeons working on my one face. It seemed to complicate not just the logistic of coordinated schedules, but surgical aftercare and accountability as well. The entire consultation didn't feel right to me. It seemed too slick, too impersonal. Somehow I just didn't feel like his heart was in it.

Several days later, I received a letter from Dr. S. . . It opened with the statement that he considered me "an exceptional candidate for facial rejuvenation". I wondered how he could make that claim without any questions directed at the state of my physical health or mental well-being. His letter ended with a detailing of his television and radio appearances. With all the time he devoted to PR, I wondered how he could devote sufficient time to keeping abreast of developments in surgical techniques and technologies and continue to hone his skills. My initial feelings of discomfort were confirmed. I crossed the Dr. S. . . /Dr. R. . . team off my list.

I went for a consultation with one of the big names in Manhattan on a Friday afternoon. He examined me ever so briefly, then stood poised with one hand on the brass knob of his examining room door as we spoke. I felt like his mind was already focused on ocean breezes and candlelight dinners rather than me, the prospective patient. Perhaps he had a weekend date in the Hamptons. I did not return for a follow-up consultation.

I confided in my friend **Carole**, my daughter-in-law's mother, that I was thinking of having a facelift. "I think I'd really like to do this for myself", I whispered, "but I'm having difficulty substantiating such an egocentric expense."

I knew I could count on Carole for a ready retort.

> "Look", she remarked. "You have longevity on your side. How old is your mother? Ninety something? I mean, if you thought you were going to die in a few years, maybe it would be an extravagance. But look at all the years you'll have to enjoy it. You could be going into the hospital, spending money on treatment for a horrible disease. Why not spend it on something to make yourself feel wonderful?"

Leave it to Carole to shake me out of my usual practicality. Money was always a non-issue to her. Then as an aside she said: "You know, we have a marvelous plastic surgeon right here in town, Dr. K. . ."

Yes, from the depths of my memory I knew that name. Dr. K. . . had reconstructed the faces of two young adults I knew, both of whom had been badly injured in accidents, unrelated by time or circumstance. Both families had raved about this marvelous plastic surgeon – his surgical skills, demeanor and most important, the results he had achieved. I just wasn't aware that he had long since dedicated his practice to *cosmetic* plastic surgery.

My next door neighbor, **Marie Gemma**, a warm hearted friend and compassionate Registered Nurse, has been my most valued resource for medical recommendations over a course of twenty plus years. She has never once steered me wrong. I asked her whom she would recommend if someone in her family wanted cosmetic surgery. Without hesitation she answered:

> Dr. K. . . - he's brilliant. I have such admiration for his surgical skills and his artistry. They are just flawless. And post-operatively, he is extremely attentive, so well mannered, so respectful of his

220

patients. When I think of him, the two words that come to mind are integrity and trust. When my son's wife was in a car accident, I didn't hesitate for a second. 'Ask for Dr. K . . .', I practically shouted into the phone."

The next day I called to schedule a consultation with Dr. K .

Two weeks later, I walked into his office, stopped at the sign-in desk and was asked to make a right turn to enter the waiting room. (I later learned that a left turn led to the area reserved for post-operative patients.) I was given a clipboard and questionnaire to complete: medical history, medications, allergies, etc. I had no medical conditions beyond my eye ptosis and little to report. My only medication was a three time weekly topical steroid for my eye, my only surgery an early childhood tonsillectomy and I had no pre-existing conditions or allergic responses to medications, I was able to complete my rather boring medical history in two minutes, leaving me with plenty of time to look around.

I glanced about the waiting room - asymmetrical in both its architectural design and its placement of furniture. The décor, tasteful and pleasing without a decorator feel. A vase of colorful, freshly cut flowers sat on an elongated table as a welcoming focal point. This room made a refined yet unpretentious statement. I liked that.

I walked over to a table with a collection of papers pertaining to Dr. K. . .'s professional contributions. As I read some of the literature, I began to discover how thoroughly immersed he was in this field of cosmetic surgery. I was impressed by his dedication and standing amongst peers, the many articles he had published in medical journals, the presentations he had made at professional conferences, his active involvement in the prestigious ASAPS.

I spotted a framed poster hanging on one wall and began to

read. It depicted two characters from Greek Mythology, with identifying text to tell the story:

The young hero, Proseus overcame the ghastly creature, Medusa by looking at her reflection in his shield. Then he decapitated her.

That prior weekend Ken and I had seen the show Cellini at the Second Stage Theatre in Manhattan, so I was newly primed on this 16th century Italian Renaissance artist who had sculpted a looming statue of Proseus. A serendipitous moment: Cellini, the Proseus poster and the man who had selected it to hang on his office wall. They all converged in my head as something more than coincidence.

I read on:

> *Don't come face to face with a ghastly schedule. Complete your registration for summer term now.*

I'll be darned! This was nothing more than a classy college campus poster reminding students to register before getting shut out of their preferred classes. No decorator art – just something that obviously held significance to this man and his life. I was feeling a sense of connection before we even met.

Soft spoken, quietly charming, speech punctuated by a British accent born of South Africa, Dr. K. . . brings a comfort level to a first meeting that I didn't think would be possible. I felt instantly secure and at ease.

He studied my face carefully and asked me why I had come to him. What differences was I hoping to achieve.

> "Dr. K. . ., I'm still in shock that I'm thinking of doing this. I've never considered myself a particularly vain person or one to focus that much on outward appearances", I began apologetically. "But once I realized I needed eyelid surgery, I got to

thinking about doing some cosmetic work at the same time. I guess what's bothering me most is the areas above and below my eyes and the lower part of my face and neck."

Dr. K. . . lifted my chin to get a better full-face view. Then slowly he turned my head, first to the left, then to the right. He was studying. Then he extended a hand mirror for me to take a look.

"This is what I would suggest for you", he began: "Upper and lower eye lift to get rid of the extra tissue here and here (touching above my lids and the deepening rings below my eyes), a facelift to get rid of this (touching the lower portion of my face and neck) and a chin implant. Yes indeed, a chin implant will make a world of difference!"

A chin implant, I thought to myself. To be sure, the individual words chin and implant were well entrenched in my vocabulary. I just had never heard them spoken in unison before.

Dr. K. . . gracefully circumvented my open mouthed stare with a further question: "Would you like to see photographs of some of my other patients?"

At this point I was speechless, so I just nodded affirmatively. He brought forth an album of truly magnificent photographs. Beyond his other talents, he was an excellent photographer. The transformation between the before and after shots of these women was simply incredible. I was looking at well lit, non-shadowed photographs, taken in similar before and after poses, which gave a very clear presentation of his surgical skills. The results were so natural that I never would have guessed any of them had achieved their physical attractiveness through cosmetic surgery.

"These are incredible", I began as I regained my voice.

"Did you work on this woman's nose?", I continued. I was looking at the before and after photos of a handsome woman with silver gray hair. I had always considered my nose my least attractive feature, favoring little button noses that pointed north. I felt self-conscious about my profile, preferring full face or three quarter camera angles.

At first he responded with a negative, but then as an afterthought reconsidered:

"Yes, you're right, I had almost forgotten. I did a little work, but just on the tip of her nose."

"How come you never said anything about my nose?", I asked.

Dr. K. . . turned my head sideways for another look.

> "Your nose is fine. Leave your nose alone. Look, it even turns up a little at the end. Your problem isn't your nose; it's your chin. It's too recessed and causes the muscles on the sides of your mouth to pull down. See, you have an overbite. It's out of alignment with your other features."

I tend to be a little skeptical when presented with unexpected options, suspecting a sales gimmick to get me to purchase one thing more. But I didn't react that way. Instead I experienced the emergence of an ah-ha revelation.

> *How amazing!*, I thought to myself.
> *I've lived my whole life thinking my nose was too big for my face. Have I had the wrong culprit all these years? Have I been unjustifiably hard on my nose, when it's really my chin that's to blame?*

"How much would this all cost?", I asked.

He spoke the numbers in such an upfront manner. I loved his honesty. "You can sit down with Anne (pronounced Annie) after we finish and she'll print it all out for you. My advice: Do it all or don't bother with any of it."

Then I asked my question:

"Dr. K. . . , if I do all that you recommend, do you think there would be a dramatic, moderate or slight difference in my overall appearance?"

He smiled kindly, eyes twinkling as he nodded his head up and down.

"You will like it", he said simply.

As soon as I arrived home, I picked up a hand mirror and headed for my bedroom. I angled that mirror so I could get a good profile reflection in the mirror on my bathroom wall. Then I cupped my left hand around my lower face, trying to envision a bit more prominent chin. Dr. K. . . was right. My chin was throwing off the balance of my face. Not only was I amazed by this revelation, but I felt a rush of excitement at the thought of defeating the ravages of age and outsmarting Mother Nature in one swoop.

Next I went to Dr. K's . . .website, which confirmed my impressions. There was no glitter - no seductive silhouette of a naked woman, just an impressive array of credentials to catch my eye:

"a nationally renowned cosmetic surgeon . . . (with a) unique artistic vision and advanced clinical skills. . . a talented, expertly trained cosmetic surgeon, (Dr. K. . .) has been obtaining beautiful, natural results for his patients for nearly 30 years. His outstanding surgical skills, welcoming bedside manner, and extensive experience have not only earned him recognition from his professional peers, but they have also made him a popular choice for patients seeking a safe, rewarding cosmetic surgery experience.'

"Raised in Johannesburg, South Africa, he graduated from The University of the Witwatersrand and received his medical degree from the New York State Education Department. He then completed a general surgery residency and a plastic surgery residency at Mt. Sinai Hospital in New York, . . . has also worked with some of the top surgeons in the nation, including Dr. I. Jackson and Dr. Ian McGregor of Canniesburn Hospital in Glasgow . . .'

"A Fellow of the Royal College of Surgeons of Edinburgh (F.R.C.S.) and a Fellow of the American College of Surgeons (F.A.C.S.), . . ., board certified by the American Board of Plastic Surgeons, and a member of a number of reputable professional organizations. . . . A private practitioner, . . . on staff at some of the community's best hospitals, including Huntington Hospital in Huntington (where he is chief of plastic surgery), Stony Brook University Hospital in Stony Brook, and North Shore University Hospital in Manhasset.'

"A notable author, lecturer, and teacher, Dr. K. . . is an assistant professor of plastic surgery at Stony Brook University Hospital and has published articles on a wide array of topics, such as microdermabrasion and endoscopic surgery, in a number of well respected medical journals."

I knew I had found my plastic surgeon and never looked back.

That night Ken and I talked:

"I can't understand why you would want to put yourself through all that, he said. Forget the money for a minute, it just seems so unnecessary."

I tried to explain how I was feeling . . . how I thought it would make me feel. It was hard. I didn't quite fully understand it myself, but I knew the chin implant was a big factor pushing me forward, something I wanted even more than the facelift. Ken must have felt my sense of urgency.

"Look, all I want is for you to be happy. For my children and grandchildren to be happy", he said. "If you're happy, then I'm happy too."

How I loved him at that moment. What a leap of faith for someone who couldn't even begin to understand this sudden sense of yearning.

The next morning I called Dr. K. . .'s office and asked to speak with Anne (pronounced Annie). "Anne, this is Lois Stern", I spoke into the receiver. "I'm going to go for it, but I need to do this before I lose my nerve. How soon can you work me into Dr. K. . .'s schedule?"

Miraculously, they had just gotten a call for a postponement. There was an opening on Feb. 5th, just 19 days away. Less than three weeks until a new me.

Upheavals and Preparations

My internist called me eight days before my scheduled surgery with some nerve rattling news. He planned to call Dr. K . . .to discuss whether it might be preferable to postpone my somewhat elective surgery. Test results from my required pre-surgical examination had shown an elevated white cell count, indicative of some type infection.

During those next few days, I began to unravel at the seams: broke a favorite casserole dish, missed a scheduled appointment, puddled up with tears during a phone call. It was the uncertainty that was getting to me and it took several more days and a few more tests before I got final clearance. Monday morning surgery would take place as planned. With that confirmation I was able to relax a bit, shift gears and busy myself with the domestic details I wanted to accomplish during those last two pre-surgery days.

I cooked a big pot of turkey frame soup, blended all the vegetables until smooth and poured double portions into small, freezer safe containers. I colored my hair, even though I had done so less than two weeks earlier, because I knew otherwise I would have to wait two to three more weeks to allow time for my scalp stitches to heal. I got my hair cut and blown dry, shopped for some soft and quick dissolving foods, (e.g. oatmeal, apple sauce, Oysterettes, cottage cheese, canned peaches and protein shakes). I bought a bunch of fresh tulips to perk me up.

What I thought I needed now was a grandchildren fix so I invited Jessica age 6, and Nicholas age 5 for an overnighter. Ken hunkered down in our family room to encourage the children to bury him under mounds of pillows, afghans and clothes. They were all giggles and screams. My ears began to ring from the commotion. I felt like a wind up toy whose key had been tightened one notch too far. I disappeared upstairs to retrieve my sewing machine and worked to reattach a fringe that had been yanked off a bedroom window shade. It had been sitting that way for nearly six months, but I had a sudden urge to fix it right then.

On Saturday morning, I kissed the children goodbye; then tended to some other details for a good part of that day and the next. Late Sunday afternoon, I sat down to record my first journal entry:

> "This morning I started the new regime of antibiotics prescribed by Dr. K . . .. Then I vacuumed the house with a frenzy before I left to visit Mom at her nursing home residence with a scoop of her favorite Haagen Dazs ice cream. I tried to awaken her, first just by stroking her cheeks and talking to her, then by smoothing some almond scented lotion on her hands and face. She continued to sleep. I kissed her gently and left, ice cream in tow. I stopped at the library to check out a few audio books on tape, which I thought might hold my interest during the first few post surgery days. My daily mantra: *plan ahead, keep busy, stay calm*, helped a little."

When I returned home, Ken took some varied close up shots
of me as I sat on our glassed in sun porch.

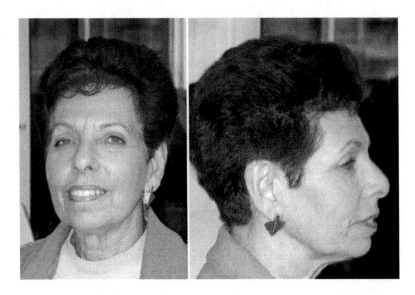

No sooner had I put away the camera then Harriet and Joel
W. stopped by to wish me luck before my big day. Joel
expressed some concern about his forthcoming visit to his
Dad, a thought which vividly yet distortedly resurfaces in my
dream early next morning. We hugged goodbye and Harriet
handed me a beautifully wrapped gift with firm instructions
not to open it for two weeks. (It turned out to be a gorgeous
aqua enameled purse size mirror.)

Ken and I started downtown for some Chinese food.

He was unusually quiet as we sat down to eat.

"Are you nervous?", I asked.
"Of course I'm nervous", he answered. "I just hate to see you
put yourself through this." At this point, I was thinking the
same thought. "What am I getting myself into? Why?"

So we talked about mundane things: that I would sleep in our
guestroom, that I planned to cover those bedroom mirrors so

I didn't have to see myself, that I had already slipped the mirrors out of the medicine chest in the guest bath. Ken suggested that I put my nightgown and fresh underwear in the guestroom as well. "If you have to walk into our bedroom, it's going to be too tempting. You'll end up looking in those mirrors, even though you don't want to."

I decided to follow his advice.

Although I opted to go undercover - no mirrors in my bedroom or bathroom – **Cookie Levy**, Dr. K. . .'s most senior Registered Nurse, has since told me this is not a good idea. "When people can see their daily progress, it encourages them and actually helps with their recovery", she explained. I have now bowed to her expertise and advise you against following my lead here.

That evening my anesthesiologist called.

He told me all about his own chin implant . . ., how much he loved it, how it had changed his life. He was so reassuring. He explained a bit more about the Twilight Sleep:

> "You'll be breathing on your own. When you wake up, you won't remember anything. You'll be thrilled with the result." I told him I was scared.

> "Of course you are", he answered. "You feel like you are giving up control and that's scary. You are about to place yourself completely into someone else's hands. But you are in excellent hands. Now you need to have faith and trust the people you selected to do this work on you."

I thought that was good advice.

The newest weather forecast spoke of six to eight inches of snow, starting before rush hour in the morning. Just what we needed, an early morning blizzard! Ken moved his car to the foot of the driveway, in case they were right. I watched some TV, which absorbed me for an hour. Then I picked up the paper, but couldn't get further than an article on genetic cloning in the magazine section of the NY Times. Ken began to peel an orange. I rarely snack after dinner, but suddenly I felt pangs of hunger as I looked at that orange. It was now 12:30 AM. No more food or drinks allowed after midnight. I went to bed without satisfying that urge.

I slept fitfully during the night. In one dream I watched in horror as my friend Joel chased his dad around his Florida apartment with a broom. I had once read that one should try to key into immediate feelings upon awakening from a dream – for it is those feelings, rather that the actual content of the dream, that are most significant. I was feeling absolutely frenetic from the chase. I knew from whence those feelings came. Simply put, I was momentarily paralyzed with fear. I would have sworn that two over-wound springs were clutching at the junctures of my upper and lower jaws, just below each ear lobe.

When terror began to creep inside me, I did two little visualization tricks that seemed to calm me. First I pictured my surgeon and kept my thoughts focused on his capable hands and gentle manner. My anesthesiologist's words:

". . . you are in excellent hands; now you need to have faith and trust the people you selected to do this work on you. . .", redirected my thoughts to where they needed to be - a sense of trust and confidence in my doctor. This is key.

Then I tried to visualize the new me, the one with fewer wrinkles and a chin prominent enough to balance my other features. That was such a helpful focus for me – to redirect my thoughts to a positive outcome.

Day of Surgery

It's Monday morning, Feb. 5th. I shake myself awake, open my left eye just a slit to glance at the clock on my night table. The small hand is slightly past the five. I realize that Ken is already awake, taking a shower in the guest bathroom. This can't be easy for him either. I turn on a light and pick up the packet I had received from Dr. K . . .'s office: *Surgical Instructions for Face Lift Surgery*. I reread it for the eleventh time.

Why am I so scared? First, it's the idea of having a scalpel cut into my face. I think of that beautiful Manhattan model whose face was slashed unmercifully by a stalker several years back. Just as quickly I suppress that thought. I try to visualize Dr. K. . .'s gentle touch and reassuring manner. That comforts me.

I wonder how I'll behave while I'm in that Twilight Sleep. Will I be prattling on in non-stop, uncensored speech or just be out of it altogether? I have to put myself in their capable hands and, as advised, give up control – totally abandon control. This is nearly as frightening to me as the image of the knife.

I take a deep breath and exhale slowly. I do this several more times. Then I get up and take a last look in the mirror. *Goodbye, old face*, I say to that image staring back at me. My fear is tinged with excitement over the thought of seeing the new me.

By 6:20 AM the beginning traces of snow are on the ground. I shower and dress in easy-to-exit clothes: a cotton knit shirt with front Velcro tabs, velour sweatpants and a matching snap up jacket, comfortable walking shoes. I brace myself for the day ahead.

I hear Ken 's footsteps coming downstairs, but it's strangely a far away sound. My ears feel like they are filled with fluid – somewhat the way they felt when I was a child, after a dive into the lake at summer camp. Suddenly I remember my plan to photographically document my daily post surgery progress and rush down our basement steps to retrieve fresh film from our spare refrigerator.

When we arrive at Dr. K. . .'s office, **Linda Gottlieb,** a Nurse Practitioner, gives me a reassuring smile, guides me to the rear O.R. center and asks me to trade in my jacket and shirt for a soft pink surgical gown. There's a drumbeat pounding in my chest. My throat feels like it's filled with cotton – dry and tasteless. I sit on a padded chair, saying aloud: "Oh, my God, what am I doing here? Why am I doing this?" I think any minute I might bolt from the room. **Linda's** calm, gentle manner sooths me. She just stroked my arm and says, "Don't worry, Lois, you're going to do just fine."

Dr. K. . . enters, greets me with the warmth of a good friend and takes some more photos unadorned by makeup. He then sets about the task of marking the areas of my face highlighted for surgery with a fine line bluish marker. It feels like he's drawing all over my face. I wonder if this is a foreshadowing of how much surgery is in store for me.

After he leaves, I look in the mirror. I see war paint around my eyes, at the frown lines on my forehead, in the creases on either side of my mouth. "What about my jowls and neck?" I ask **Linda**. "He didn't put any marks there. He won't forget them, will he?"

She assures me that those parts are too obvious for him to overlook.

A few minutes later my anesthesiologist bursts through the door like a freshly popped bottle of champagne. He pulls a somewhat crumpled photo from his pocket and thrusts it into my lap. It reflects the pre-surgical profile view of a man with a markedly recessed chin, in contrast to the strong chinned man standing before me. He talks amicably, explaining that he is about to insert a catheter into a vein in my left wrist – just something to relax me. I can't argue with that one. That catheter was the last thing I remembered. Apparently, whatever was in that IV had done its job.

About 2:45 PM Ken got the call he was awaiting. Surgery was complete. I was being taken to recovery.

It's now nearly 6:00 PM. I hear far away voices calling my name. I just can't focus or open my eyes. It takes my supreme effort to follow even the simplest command, like: *Lois, open your eyes.* Two nurses are smiling down at me. They work as a team to help me sit me up and get dressed and then support my weight as they guide me into a standing position. With one arm draped over each of their shoulders, I shuffle my way with tiny baby steps as they walk me around the room, through the hall and out the back door. It is dark out by now. Sleet is coming down with a vengeance.

My head is swathed in a helmet-like wrapping of bandages. I see Ken standing beside our car, waiting nervously. He helps guide me into my seat on the passenger side and buckles my seat belt. **Rosalie Cropper**, my private duty nurse, trails closely behind. Two minutes on the road and Ken emits an expletive. His driver side windshield wiper has snapped. Now we have to contend not only with icy roads, but obscured vision as well.

It was a stressful ride home. Ken was trying to peer between the sleety snowflakes falling in increasingly rapid succession. The roads were covered with an icy snow. The broken wiper was doing an inadequate job of clearing the windshield. After riding for what seemed much too long, Ken stopped at a corner and got out of the car to read the street sign. He had gone way past the turn to our street. Lost in the neighborhood where we have lived for over 30 years!

Ken finally pulls our car into the garage and waits for **Rosalie** to enter the driveway behind us. The two of them help me up the basement steps to the kitchen and then up a second flight to the guest bedroom upstaris. I am prone to stress headaches under ordinary circumstances, so I wasn't surprised to feel one beginning to surface at that moment.

Rosalie takes charge. First she takes my blood pressure: 142 over 101.

"I might have to call Dr. K. . . ", she says. "It's pretty high, but that might be because of the ride home and the two flights of steps you just climbed to get upstairs. We'll take it again in a few minutes." Dr. K. . . called several minutes later to check on how I was doing. My blood pressure had already stabilized. Rosalie briefed him on everything, including the details of our slippery trek home in the storm. Oh, how I wished at that moment that Dr. K . . .'s recovery suite, then under construction, had been ready for me that evening!

Now Rosalie goes into full action, placing zip lock bags filled with frozen peas over the rolled towels adjacent to the helmet dressing on either side of my face. She lays iced gauze pads over my eyelids. She continues to make me comfortable: two pillows under my head and a third pillow under my legs, two Tylenol gel caps for my headache. I guess that helped a little. I remember between icings taking Rosalie for a tour of the other bedrooms and being somewhat amazed that I actually felt well enough to talk and walk around.

By 10:00 o'clock my headache has returned – stronger than before. I wish I could take some Excedrin. I know that would help, but also know that it is forbidden due to its aspirin content. **Rosalie** gives me one Darvocet tablet for the pain, but it doesn't seem to do much good. I feel pressure on the back of my head. Somehow, I just can't get comfortable flat on my back, propped by two pillows. I take frequent sips of water through a flexible straw.

Meanwhile, Rosalie continues applying ice packs and zip lock bags of frozen peas – fifteen minutes on and fifteen minutes off - occasionally opening the zip lock bags to air out the peas. "They get smelly after awhile, but they work so well", she says as she explains the merits of frozen peas. I learn that they conform to all facial contours, don't leak and can be refrozen and used again.

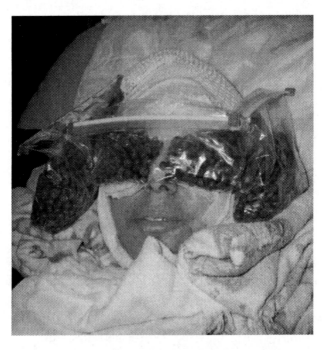

She heats up some of the turkey frame pureed vegetable soup I had previously cooked and frozen and serves it to me with Oysterettes. I could just manage to open my mouth wide enough to accommodate a child size spoon.

Stacey Lanza, the second shift nurse, arrives on schedule at 11:00 PM and Rosalie briefs her before we say good-bye. **Stacey** takes over with the same competence and efficiency. My vision is still quite blurred from the ointment in my eyes, but through the glaze I see a young, pretty face and a slightly pregnant body. She entertains me with funny tales she has heard in her travels. My favorite was the one about the fifty-eight year old woman who was terrified of her impending facelift, not because of the surgery but because of her husband. In their eighteen years of marriage, they had never missed a beat in their sex lives. It was a nightly event, even when she had the flu. How would she ever keep him at bay? Her surgeon had to sit her husband down for a serious chat, advising him that this kind of post surgery activity was verboten. At worst, it could be life threatening. At best, it would most definitely interfere with his wife's healing. This middle aged marathon man was compelled to break his Olympian record.

As the ointment began to clear from my eyes, I noticed a red blob on the dresser. I blinked and refocused - a vase of two dozen red roses from Ken with the simple message: *I love you.* What a sweetheart!

Day One Post Surgery

I sleep on and off, not for any solid block of time, and yet I don't feel tired. My headache continues unabated as does the feeling of pressure at the back of my head. At 7:00 AM I say good-bye to Stacey.

Ken begins his stay-at-home duty by bagging more frozen peas. He makes enough ice cubes to build an igloo. He experiments with different icing systems as he covers my whole face with a hand towel and strategically places ice bags on my neck and cheeks, zip lock bags of frozen peas over my eyes. The towel acts as a buffer between my skin

237

and the chill. He cooks me oatmeal for breakfast and heats up more of that delicious soup with Oysterettes for lunch. I sit like a lump, dozing on and off, accepting all the help that Ken offers.

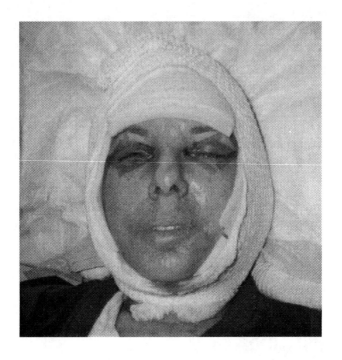

At 3:15 we return to Dr. K . . .'s office for my first follow-up appointment.

Linda removes my helmet dressing. 'Wow! You look great!", she enthuses.

When Dr. K . . . enters the room he seems truly delighted with the results of his handiwork. "You look super. Have you looked at yourself yet?", he asks.
I tell him I'm afraid – that I covered all the mirrors in my house so I don't have to look.

"No, I want you to look. You look wonderful", he says as he extends a hand mirror.

With his reassurance, I take a peek. What do I see? My skin appears taut and smooth. The vertical lines between my brows and on either side of my mouth – GONE! My face is puffy, with some bruising under my eyes and on my cheeks, but not nearly as much as I had anticipated. My neck is another story. Its circumference could easily match that of a Heisman Trophy winner. It is bejeweled by a choke collar necklace formed from a continuous band of deep purple bruises. This might sound like a formidable sight, but I was already thrilled with the results.

"Wow! This is amazing, I didn't think I would look so good so soon", I say.

"I used something called tissue glue in parts of your surgery, explained Dr. K . . . . It's fairly new, but I've been finding that it cuts down on the amount of swelling and bruising. I only use it in special situations. I needed to do a lot of cutting on you."

I inquire about tissue glue and learn that it is considered quite safe because it is formed by a mixture of coagulants from the patient's own blood. Dr. K . . . tells me that this fibrant sealant has been used in general surgery for over twenty years, but only recently for cosmetic procedures. He explains that ordinarily, after being cut, the body adheres to itself as it creates its own form of fibrin glue. But this takes time. With the spray adhesive, the tissue adheres immediately, so patients experience less swelling and bruising. Another advantage is that post surgery drains are not needed. He tells me that its only down side is its high cost, - about $500 per surgery. I later learn that there is a further down side to tissue glue. Because it sets so quickly, the surgeon needs to 'get it right' the first time. This makes for a strong learning curve before one can use it effectively, but Dr. K . . never mentions this.

As soon as we return home, I dart upstairs, headed straight for our master bathroom. I grab my hand mirror, open the medicine cabinet, to reveal more mirrors inside, then lock the bathroom door to assure my privacy. I want to relish this magical moment as I angle mirrors in various positions to reflect my post surgical being. I must familiarize myself with this new person – this person I like on contact, but need to get to know more intimately.

The disappearance of lines and wrinkles, the brightness of my eyes, the smoothness of my neck - all of these contribute to my pleasure. It feels great to see a refreshed version of myself. But it is my chin that catches most of my focus. While my facelift makes me feel renewed, it is my chin that makes me feel like a new version of myself.

I cringe ever so slightly as I think back to my teenage years. All those times when I entered a theatre with my date of the moment, how I would maneuver to remain face to face rather than in profile view – that is, until the very last second when the lights were ready to dim. My strategy was clear – to shield my date from a side view of my nose, that self-appointed culprit to my marred good looks. Little did I realize that I would have had equal success with less maneuvering had I simply posed like Rodin's 'Thinker', with my hand resting up against my chin. It was my new chin that made me feel not just younger, but prettier as well.

Again Dr. K . . .'s words came back to me: *You should have done this years ago.* Did he know that a new chin would have such an emotional impact or was he thinking purely of aesthetic harmony? Either way, he was right.

After dinner, Ken is on schedule with repeated icings to my face and neck. It seems like my skin is just about returning to room temperature when we begin again. Now that my gauze helmet headgear has been removed, he devises a new system: one presoaked large size gauze pad stretched from the outer bridge of the nose, across the right eyelid and over the right ear. A second gauze pad extended similarly leftward. Zip lock bags of frozen peas covering both eyes, zip lock bags of crushed ice over my cheeks, neck and jaw. It seemed to work just fine, and cut down on set-up time.

At bedtime, I place a couch bolster on either side of me so that I don't roll over in my sleep. Now I'm on my own. I keep a cooler of ice water on the floor nearby along with a fresh supply of gauze pads. I soak each pad in the ice water and spread it over a different part of my face or neck. I do this again at about 1:30 AM. Finally I fall asleep but awaken after several hours.

Day Two Post Surgery

"My head feels like it's the weight of a bowling ball", I say to Ken when he peaks in my room the next morning. "I feel like I need a pillow that's hollowed out in the center to relieve some of the pressure."

Ken decides to take another day off. This wasn't preplanned, but I don't complain. I'm happy to have him home with me. He continues keeping his charts of times for medication and icings. He decides today we will move to a half hour on, half hour off schedule for ice soakings. I ask for a double thickness of pads to cover my ears, which are numb yet tender. I wonder how they can be both things at once.

I spend most of the day in my recliner chair: icing, thawing, reading (at least the lead stories in the NY Times), dozing and writing in my journal. I examine my scalp in the mirror and see three vertical rows of stitches, some of which continue downward both within and behind my ears. The stitches on my eyelids are considerably lighter.

I defrost homemade turkey croquettes and spaghetti for dinner and am delighted to discover that I am actually able to eat without first removing the crunchy outer crust from the croquettes.

I sleep intermittently throughout the night. Physically I feel pretty good. My headache is dull, but annoying, my right ear totally numb, the sides of my face, semi-numb and still somewhat swollen. As for my neck, well, let's forget about my neck right now. It needs a lot of healing.

Day Three Post Surgery

I shower, dress and eat a softly scrambled egg. I don a large scarf and sunglasses before Ken and I set off for my 9:30 AM post-surgical appointment.

Linda removes the stitches on my upper and lower eyelids. She's very gentle but it's such a sensitive area that I wince a little. She says the scalp stitches need to remain a bit longer.

Using a syringe, Dr. K. . . removes some of the clear fluid which has accumulated beneath my left cheek and on the right side of my Heisman Trophy-sized-neck and advises me to keep massaging those areas. He works a halter-like bandage under my chin, across the sides of my face and finally to the top of my head to put pressure on my neck and discourage both further fluid buildup and unnecessary head movement.

He looks over my eyes and notes that the right eye, the one with Ptosis, is opened more than the left. He thinks that the muscles in my right eye are accustomed to working extra hard to keep that eye opened and suspects that it will even out in a couple of weeks. He advises a wait-and-see approach, but explained that if nature does not take its course, a simple office procedure would be all that would be necessary. It became a mute point. My eyes evened out without further intervention.

I have some upbeat moments this afternoon. I receive a beautiful floral arrangement from five colleague friends, and later speak with two of them on the phone. I can't use an ordinary phone receiver because even the slightest pressure against either ear causes discomfort. The speakerphone is a perfect solution to keep me in touch with the outside world.

My daughter-in-law, Kristen, visits with handmade cards from each of the grandchildren and gives me an enthusiastic thumbs up. I eat baked flounder and mashed potatoes for dinner and notice that it is definitely getting easier to eat, although I still feed myself with a baby spoon. Two more milestones tonight: I brush my teeth with a child size toothbrush instead of a Q-Tip and take my last prophylactic antibiotic pill prescribed by Dr. K . . .

After dinner I click into my e-mail, compose one message and cc it to a small group of friends. I thank them all for their warm thoughts and expressions of caring and tell them how much their support means to me. I say that I am actually doing quite well, am much less bruised and swollen than I had anticipated and then share a few details about my recovery. I end with:

> "Everything seems a bit better day by day. This is no stroll on the beach, but on the other hand, I can look beneath the bruises and swelling and know that I will be thrilled with the results. Would I recommend this to others? It's such an individual decision, that I'm not sure I should go out on that limb. But if anyone were so inclined, I would definitely encourage them. One day soon I will have an unveiling."

Day Four Post Surgery

My neck appears more swollen this morning. I call Dr. K . . .
's office. They advise me to come in at 10:15 AM. He again
inserts a needle into the right side of my neck to remove two
syringes full of fluid, then exerts gentle pressure to extract
more. He tells me that he is glad I called because, even
though my body would eventually absorb this fluid, (which
in medical terms is known as a seroma), it is best to get rid of
it quickly to accelerate healing. He gives me some concealer
make-up, just in case I want to go out this weekend. I don't!
I ask about the wedge shaped foam pillow recommended at
the surgical supply store, but Dr. K . . . advises against it,
explaining that it is best to lie flat on my back with my chin
pointed upward, slightly hyper extended.

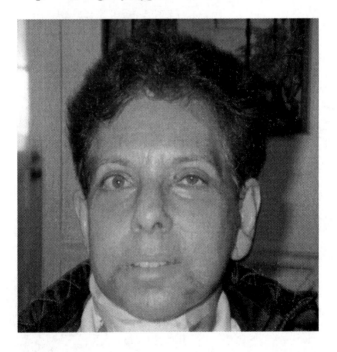

I recalled how **Rosalie** had placed a rolled washcloth under
my chin to tilt it upward and used her technique when I got
into bed that night.

Day Five Post Surgery

I'm feeling a bit more like myself, with more energy during the day and a better sleep pattern at night. Best of all, my head doesn't feel so heavy or weighted after several hours of sleep.

Day Six Post Surgery

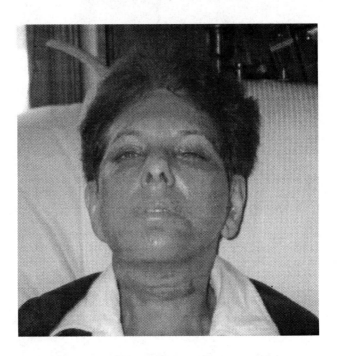

Today is the first day I feel grounded enough to tackle the notes I had been jotting into my journal. I start with an outline and proceed to a draft of a section entitled: *Who Am I?*, which keeps me occupied for several days.

I stop for lunch at 2:00 PM and nuke another bowl of soup. I have eaten all the Oysterettes, so I settle for low-salt saltine crackers. I notice that I no longer need to wait for them to dissolve in my mouth. I can actually take bites, chew and swallow. That's tangible progress. Dinner is a little more of a challenge. I cut very thin vertical slices of the salmon fillet, but need to turn each slice sideways to slip it into my mouth.

Day Seven Post Surgery

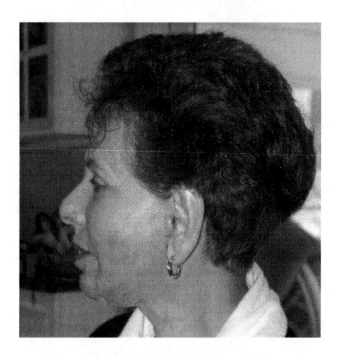

Today much of the bruising is gone from my neck, but there is still a large bruise on my left cheek.. The area in front of each ear is still pretty numb, as is my right ear. I put up a load of wash, eat breakfast and come upstairs to continue writing. I begin an outline for the next segment of my book, which I call *The Journey*.

I sleep through the night without benefit of Tylenol PM. It's not that I'm in any pain – not even real discomfort any longer - it's just a bit difficult for me to sleep flat on my back.

Day Nine Post Surgery

Today I plan my first outing and go to visit my mom at her nursing home. I hadn't seen her since the day before surgery and was eager to resume my schedule of alternate day visits. I keep a scarf around my neck, but otherwise no camouflage. Nurses and aides greet me as usual. No one acts startled by my new look.

I found Mom asleep in her Geri chair. I kissed her eyelids, stroked her cheeks and said: "Mom, can you open your eyes? I want you to look at me. I did something wonderful for myself."

To my astonishment, she did as I asked. Then I experienced my private miracle. This woman who hadn't made direct eye contact with anyone or spoken a coherent word for over five months, looked straight up at me, studied my face and said: "You look beautiful, absolutely beautiful."

Tears streamed down my cheeks as I answered her."Do you know how much I love you? How much I've always loved you?", I asked.

She smiled and spoke these next words with absolute clarity: "Well, I must have done something right."

That was the last conversation I ever had with my mom.

Day Ten Post Surgery

I call Harriet W. to see if we can meet for lunch. "You'll recognize me." I quip into the receiver. "I'll be the one with the young neck."

When we meet, she keeps hugging me and saying: "It's incredible, just incredible." I ask , "Harriet, do you really see such a change?". "Lois, are you kidding? When you go home, I want you to pull out one of your photo albums from twenty years ago. That's what you look like."

She reminds me that she had left me a gift before surgery, with strict instructions not to open it for two weeks. "I know it's early", she says. "But you are ready. Go home and open it."
I did and found the most thoughtful gift – a beautiful folding purse mirror.

Day Eleven Post Surgery

I awakened this morning with a strange sense of foreboding. Was this all a dream? Was this new look simply a figment of my imagination? The uncertainty was so unsettling that I actually jumped up and bolted to the bathroom. *Have I turned back into a frog?,* I wondered, before taking a reassuring look in the mirror.

That afternoon I'm back in the waiting room at Dr. K . . .'s office. I bring along my pre and post surgery photos from home, which the staff seems to thoroughly enjoy. Dr. K . . . is pleased with my progress, but tells me that my skin has a thick, sallow look and suggests that it would be a good idea for me to make an appointment with an esthetician to learn some better skin care techniques. I feel rebuked, like a child being blamed for something she hasn't done, but nonetheless decide to follow his advice. I leave his office with a prescription for .1% Triamcinolone Acetodide Cream and lowered exuberance.

Day Thirteen Post Surgery

I meet with **Michelle Martel**. The chemistry between us is good from the start. Aside from being an incredibly knowledgeable and skilled esthetician, she is upbeat, easy to talk with and just plain fun to be around.

"You are still healing", she explained. "We need to be very gentle right now. I don't want to do too much this soon. But I can do some things to help you heal."

She applied ultra sound and electric stimulation to the right side of my neck, the area still most tender from the surgery. Those treatments made an appreciable difference.

I had no further setbacks. Healing continued to progress without incident and my spirits soared. I learned that the path to recovery is steady, but not always smooth.

Two Months Post Surgery

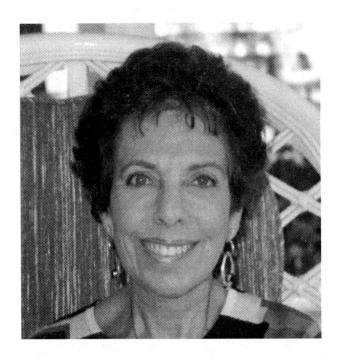

Let's now fast-forward to two months post surgery, when a day of serendipitous moments heightened my awareness of the reality of both good and poor results. These moments also reinforced my conviction that it is critically important to select your surgeon with care.

Ken and I are back at the Second Stage Theatre, waiting for a performance of Crimes of the Heart. A woman in the lobby is walking toward me. From the distance, quite stunning - long blonde hair pulled back in a carefully coiffed style, smartly tailored ebony suit, snug enough to reveal a slim, curvaceous body. As she comes a bit closer, I see something that distresses me. Her skin is pulled so taut that it has rendered her face nearly expressionless. To me it screams *facelift, bad one!* If my surgery had left me with that kind of look, I would be wearing a Muslim burqa over my head.

While Ken is getting us coffee, I walk over to a table with three seated people and two vacant seats.
"Are these seats free?", I ask.
"Oh, by all means, do join us", speaks the gentleman. In no time we are engaged in lively conversation about theatre, various productions and favorite playwrights we each enjoy. We introduce ourselves: **Stanley**, **Gladwyn**, **Edith**, **Lois** (and later) **Ken**.

All the while I am noting their accents, so reminiscent of Dr. K. . .'s speech. "Are you people from South Africa by any chance?", I finally ask.

"Why yes", they say, with some surprise.

In my present state of euphoria, I continue without a moment's forethought. "I thought so. We have a very fine plastic surgeon in our hometown on Long Island who comes from South Africa, and he sounds just like all of you."

"Oh, Alan, how do you know Alan?", asks **Gladwyn**,

referring to my plastic surgeon, Dr. Alan Kisner.

By now Ken has joined us and steps in to rescue me. "Oh, he's a friend", says Ken nonchalantly.

"Why, I don't remember meeting you at one of their parties, the man persists.

No, not that kind of friend", Ken answers.

"Oh, I see", says **Stanley**, but it's clear he is perplexed.

I can't control my amusement and start to laugh as I confess: "Well, to be quite honest, I am one of his patients."

World of coincidence or six degrees of separation? I wonder which as I learn that **Stanley** is also a plastic surgeon and personal friend of Dr. K. . . They left South Africa at about the same time for their advance surgical training at Mt. Sinai Hospital.

We talk a bit about Dr. K. . . . I tell them that I enjoy his personality:

> "In some ways he comes across as sophisticated, but then he'll come out with something that strikes me so funny – almost playful or naive. Like the day he admired my teeth and then asked me if they were mine. Or when he told me that he had heard that my husband and I were checking out real estate on our trip home after surgery. Actually we did get lost in a blinding snowstorm that evening."

"Yes, he's very boyish", laughs **Edith**.

Now we are on a roll, so I continue. "Well, Stanley, now that you know my secret, do you think Dr. K. . . did a good job?"

"He certainly did", says **Stanley**, "and I'll tell you why. I never would have known. That's the way we were trained. Not to overdo."

Stanley's simple statement confirmed what I already knew: I had chosen well.

I am ever aware that my story might have ended differently, had I not placed myself in the hands of such a capable plastic surgeon. For one thing, I wouldn't have had a chin implant. No one had recommended it and I wouldn't have even known to ask for it. Secondly, my early healing was simplified – no need for drains and far less swelling and bruising - because of the use of Tissue Glue. My plastic surgeon, a member of the Innovative Procedure Committee of the Aesthetic Surgery Education and Research Foundation (ASERF), the education and research arm of the American Society for Aesthetic Plastic Surgery (ASAPS), was familiar with the newest techniques and skilled in their use. I was the beneficiary. And finally, my end result – refreshed and renewed without a tight, *plastic* look, healed without the trace of a scar – is the result every plastic surgery candidate would hope for.

If you decide to go for cosmetic surgery, I want you to have as successful an experience. How do you know? How do you choose? Start by becoming a savvy consumer.

Helpful Resources:

For further information on topics relevant to this Epilogue, please refer to the following end-of-book Appendices:

🔔 **Appendix 4: Selecting Your Surgeon – The First Two R's**

🔔 **Appendix 5: Relaxation Techniques – Ways to Calm Your Mind**

🔔 **Appendix 8: Personal Profiles (More about the people whose names appear in this chapter)**

🔔 **Appendix 9: Additional Stories to my Epilogue**

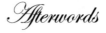

The Short Story:

A few words in closing

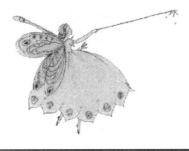

I begin this final segment with a few words about after you are healed:

♦ When a client tells **Denise Thomas** that she wants cosmetic procedures to multiple parts of her body (e.g. a facelift and a tummy tuck), Denise advices her to start with her face, because that is what people notice first. (Denise is not a proponent of having too many procedures in one surgery, despite the extremes depicted in TV surgical makeovers.) No matter what procedure you have undergone, don't forget to focus on your face. If you haven't yet learned how to care for your skin, now is a good time to start.

♦ Buy a good quality Sunscreen to use on a daily basis throughout the year – no exceptions. (Look for a screen with Zinc Oxide or Titanium Dioxide listed as its first ingredient. There are a number of excellent sunscreens on the market. *The Duchess of Dermis*, **Michelle Martel**, introduced me to a

Topix product called Citrix Antioxidant Sunscreen SPF 30, containing healthy antioxidants and 7% zinc oxide, compounded in such micronized particles that it doesn't leave your skin with a white masked look.

♦ Hydrate your skin from the inside out. Drink plenty of water throughout the day, every day. I store several thirty-two ounce plastic bottles filled with filtered water in my refrigerator and start each day by placing one of them in an insulated bottle bag with an over the shoulder strap. I tote it with me wherever I go: upstairs to my office, in the car, to meetings and informal gatherings. Sipping water throughout the day has become part of my daily routine for general good health and healthier skin.

♦ Exercise. Once you get into an exercise routine, you will want to stick with it because not only will you *feel* healthier, but you will in fact *be* healthier, both physically and mentally. Physical fitness is to our bodies what fine tuning is to our automobiles; it enables our heart, lungs and muscles to perform closer to their potential. Fitness also impacts our mental alertness and emotional stability. Finally, there is an aesthetic component to exercise. As your body becomes firmer and better toned, you will look better too. Exercise sets in motion a cycle of psychic enhancements, which begins with our physical appearance, but ultimately also impacts our health and self-esteem.

You have to find the routine that works best for you. I am an early riser and like to open my eyes, throw on an oversize T shirt and jump on my treadmill. I run on the treadmill for forty minutes at least five times a week. I put on earphones and play disco music, which automatically quickens my stride. After I rest just a little, but not long enough for my body to cool down, I exercise with weights - on alternate days, doing routines for upper or lower body fitness. Occasionally I have a personal trainer come to my home to monitor and diversify my program. Many women prefer the structure of a gym. You have to do what fits your comfort level and lifestyle.

♦ Find a knowledgeable esthetician and engage her services. I once thought of the use of an esthetician as an unnecessary extravagance, but now appreciate their value. If you have had cosmetic work done on your face, think of your esthetician as the protector of your investment. **Michelle** and I started with the basics such as *How do you cleanse your face?*, and she nearly exploded when I told her I used whatever bar of soap happened to be in my shower. I had a lot to learn. She started me on a skin care routine with just the right products for my skin type. After cleansing with Cetaphil lotion, I apply a toner followed by Citrix CRS 20% Cell Rejuvenation Serum and sunscreen every morning. In the evening, I cleanse similarly, but then use Albolene Moisturizing Cleanser or a moisture pad to remove all traces of make-up. (You might be surprised to see what comes off on those pads after you think you have cleansed so thoroughly.) Twice a week I use Replenix Fortified Exfoliation Scrub and again apply the same Cell Rejuvenation Serum I use each morning - both made by Topix Pharmaceuticals, Inc. I never had a beautiful complexion, but now, when I get compliments about my appearance, people comment on my skin first.

You can schedule appointments with an esthetician to suit your budget. Even an appointment once every several months can generate good results. Just exercise care in selecting your esthetician as you did with your surgeon. You want someone who is knowledgeable, skilled, experienced, comes highly recommended from people with visibly good results and has a passion for what she does. Then follow her advice.

I was intrigued to discover that in her book, *Face Value*, the cosmetic dermatologist, Dr. Hema Sundaram, recommends an earlier generation of the same Topix products that Michelle has made part of my daily routine.

That said, I would like to end with a quote from the president of Barnard College, spoken during a recent commencement address:

> "The pursuit of liberal learning involves a search for truths, a respect for facts, a healthy skepticism, an openness to criticism, and a willingness to test ideas and theories. If you have reason to consider your views well founded, you stand by them, even in the face of opposition, and you seek to persuade others of their merits. And conversely, if you hear a better argument, you are able to let go of your own, changing your mind and your approach." **1**

Perhaps it is because I am a graduate of Barnard College that I have taken this philosophy with me in life and have certainly lived it in the writing of this book. I knew my experiences with cosmetic surgery were just that, my experiences, one woman's story. They might have made for somewhat interesting reading, but I doubted that my individual experiences merited a book - unless they matched those of other women. If so, I had uncovered some truths not yet spoken about women and cosmetic surgery. If not, if there was no match between my experiences and those of other women, I would have been well advised to remain silent. But I suspected otherwise and began to investigate my suspicions. This book took hold only when I got enough confirming evidence.

I have the greatest regard for the field of plastic surgery, with its many brilliant, highly skilled professionals in possession of artistic vision and passion for their work. But when it comes to emotions and feelings surrounding cosmetic surgery, the real experts are the women who have undergone cosmetic procedures and the nurses and estheticians who work along with them. I am ever mindful of **Michelle's** words:

Remember, plastic surgeons are tailors of the skin, not guardians of the soul.

I know that she is right. We, as women, are the true guardians of our own souls. And each woman who has contributed to this book is an integral part of this guardianship.

Have a safe, healthy and beautiful life.

CR80

"If you have a Cosmetic Surgery story to share, please visit my website at www.sexliesandcosmeticsurgery.com where we can meet and possibly chat. I will continue to post your stories online and look forward to 'speaking' with you.

My very best,
Lois

Lois W. Stern

$\mathcal{Helpful\ Resources:}$

🔔 **Appendix 8: Personal Profiles**
(More about the people whose
names appear in this chapter)

$\mathcal{Footnotes:}$

1. President Judith Shapiro's Commencement Address, Barnard College. (Summer 2004).

The Sex, Lies and Cosmetic Surgery Forms

All ten of the *Sex, Lies and Cosmetic Surgery* forms which follow are also available in CD format at: http://www.sexliesandcosmeticsurgery.com/ or by using the mail-in coupon on Page 384 at the end of this book.

	Page
Part A: Test Your Sexuality	262
Part B: Test Your Self-Esteem	266
Part C: Self-assessment: Are You a Good Candidate For Cosmetic Surgery?	269
Part D: A Checklist: The Classic Signs of Depression	272
Part E: Get Answers to These Questions <u>Before</u> You Schedule a Consultation	275
Part F: Get Answers to These Questions <u>During</u> Your Consultation	279
Part G: The Third R: Personal Response - Rate Your Reaction to a Consultation	284
Part H: Getting Ready – Timeline Checklists	287
Part I: Test Your Body Image	296
Part J: A Body Dysmorphic Disorder (BDD) Checklist	298

CD Part A

Test Your Sexuality

The statements listed below, taken from the Snell Sexuality Scale, describe certain attitudes toward human sexuality. As such, there are no right or wrong answers, only personal responses. See ⚘ note at the end of Part A.

Instructions

For each of the three sections that follow, use the value score provided to decide the number that best indicates how strongly each statement describes your feelings about yourself. Write that number on the line in front of each statement.

When you complete each section, add your number score for that section and write that number on the Total Score line at the end of that segment.

👄 **Sexual Esteem:**

7: Strongly agree
6: Mostly agree
5: Slightly agree
4: Neither agree nor disagree
3: Slightly disagree
2: Mostly disagree
1: Strongly disagree.

___ **1.** I am a good sexual partner.

___ **2.** I would rate my sexual skill quite highly.

___ **3.** I feel good about my sexuality.

___ **4.** I am better at sex than most other people.

___ **5.** I derive pleasure and enjoyment from sex.

___**6.** I am confident about myself as a sexual partner.

___**Total Sexual Esteem Score**

👄 Sexual Focus:

7: **Strongly agree**
6: **Mostly agree**
5: **Slightly agree**
4: **Neither agree nor disagree**
3: **Slightly disagree**
2: **Mostly disagree**
1: **Strongly disagree**

___ **1.** I think about sex all the time.

___ **2.** I think about sex more than anything else.

___ **3.** Thinking about sex makes me happy.

___ **4.** I tend to be preoccupied with sex.

___ **5.** I am constantly thinking about having sex.

___ **6.** I frequently fantasize about having sex.

___**Total Sexual Focus Score**

Sexual Disappointment:

7: Strongly agree
6: Mostly agree
5: Slightly agree
4: Neither agree nor disagree
3: Slightly disagree
2: Mostly disagree
1: Strongly disagree

___ **1.** I am depressed about the sexual aspects of my life.

___ **2.** I am disappointed about the quality of my sex life.

___ **3.** I feel down about my sex life.

___ **4.** I feel unhappy about my sexual relationships.

___ **5.** I feel sad when I think about my sexual experiences.

___ **6.** I am discouraged about the sexual aspects of my life.

___**Total Sexual Disappointment Score**

How to Interpret Your Scores

Write your sexual _esteem_ score here. ___

Interpretation of Your Sexual _Esteem_ Score

42 – 37 = Compared with other women, you have very strong sexual esteem.
36 – 33 = Compared with other women, you have generally good sexual esteem.
32 – 28 = Compared with other women, your sexual esteem could use some strengthening.
27 – 24 = Compared with other women, your sexual esteem is below average.
23 or below = Your sexual esteem is lower than that of most women.

Write your sexual <u>focus</u> score here. ___

☞ **Interpretation of Your Sexual <u>Focus</u> Score:**

> **42 - 36 =** Your focus on sexual thoughts is decidedly stronger than that of most other women.
> **35 - 29 =** Compared with other women, your focus on sexual thoughts is above average.
> **28 - 24 =** Your sexual focus is about average that of other women.
> **23 – 21 =** You think about sex somewhat less than the average woman.
> **20 or below =** You think about sex considerably less than most women.

Write your sexual <u>disappointment</u> score here. ___

☞ **Interpretation of Your Sexual <u>Disappointment</u> Score:**

> **6 – 10 =** You are quite happy with the sexual aspects of your life.
> **11 – 15 =** You are happier than the average woman about the sexual aspects of your life.
> **16 – 23 =** You are about as happy as the average woman about the sexual aspects of your life.
> **24 – 32 =** You are less happy than the average woman about the sexual aspects of your life.
> **33 or higher =** You are very disappointed about the sexual aspects of your life.

For more information on sexuality, see Dr. Snell's online books at:
http://www4.semo.edu/snell/TESTING.HTM
http:////csti-cia.semo.edu/snell/books/sexuality/sexuality.htm

🖑 NOTE: A longer version of this test, with separate scoring for men and women, can be found at:
> hksrch.com.hk/quiz/sexuality2.htm
> (Do <u>not</u> use http:// for this address.)

CD Part B

Test Your Self Esteem

This printable checklist has eighteen statements pertaining to self-esteem.

Instructions

To rate your self-esteem, use the following seven point value scale to decide how much each statement relates to your feelings about yourself. Write the value score for each statement on the line preceding its number.

7: Strongly agree

6: Mostly agree

5: Slightly agree

4: Neither agree nor disagree

3: Slightly disagree

2: Mostly disagree

1: Strongly disagree.

_____ 1. I take care of my appearance by grooming carefully and dressing in becoming clothes.

_____ 2. I feel confidant of my abilities.

_____ 3. I am comfortable in my daily interactions with other women.

_____ 4. I am comfortable in my daily interactions with other men.

_____ 5. I generally feel happy and content.

_____ 6. I generally eat a healthy diet and control my weight.

_____ 7. I am comfortable when I meet new people.

_____ 8. I maintain warm relationships with friends.

_____ 9. I maintain warm relationships with family members.

_____ 10. I am willing to undertake activities that might draw attention to myself.

_____ 11. I have feelings of self-worth and personal adequacy as I go about my daily life.

_____ 12. I am willing to take risks without fear failure.

_____ 13. I usually make direct eye contact when I interact with others.

_____ 14. When someone disagrees with my point of view, I can generally enter into open discussion without anger or volatile debate.

_____ **15**. I get much satisfaction from personal accomplishments in my work or other pursuits.

_____ **16**. I take good care of my body by exercising regularly (at least two to three times a week), and I do not smoke or abuse alcohol or other drugs.

_____ **17**. Emotionally, I am generally on an even keel rather than experiencing frequent emotional roller coaster rides.

_____ **18**. I have at least one hobby or special interest which gives me considerable satisfaction.

_____ **TOTAL SCORE SELF-ESTEEM SCORE**

⚷ How to Interpret Your Score

126 - 117 = Very strong self-esteem
116 - 99 = Generally good self-esteem
98 - 81 = Self-esteem could use some
strengthening
80 - 63 = Below average self-esteem
62 or below = Low self-esteem (Needs
serious work)

You can order all ten of these *Sex, Lies and Cosmetic Surgery* printable forms in CD format at:
http://www.sexliesandcosmeticsurgery.com/
or by using the mail-in coupon at the end of this book.

CD Part C

Are You a Good Candidate for Cosmetic Surgery?

➤ **Do you have a medical condition, such as a bleeding, liver or kidney disorder, that might complicate a surgical outcome?**

> If your internist or other specialist who oversees your specific medical condition has advised you against elective surgery, yet you are still determined, consult with two well-qualified plastic surgeons and heed their advice. (But don't go shopping for that one surgeon who will say what you want to hear, because you will surely find one willing to take those risks!)

➤ **For optimum cosmetic surgery results, it is wise to first prepare your body physically.**

> Good health, reasonably appropriate weight, well-toned skin and a physically fit body all contribute to a successful outcome. Remember: cosmetic surgery is elective, not emergency surgery. Keep everything in perspective. Your health and well being come first.

➤ **If you are seriously considering cosmetic surgery, read this next question and record your answer below.**

> *What is it about my face or body that I see as a flaw or a sign of aging that concerns me?*

Every prospective cosmetic surgery candidate should be able to readily articulate a specific concern about her physical appearance.

If you answered this question specifically and effortlessly and have been given medical clearance for your surgery, continue with the self-assessment quiz that follows.

Please understand that "Yes" answers do not necessarily mean that you should not consider cosmetic surgery, but they can help you do some self-exploration before you sign on the dotted line.

1. Have you had plastic surgery before on the same area of your face or body?
___Yes ___ No

2. Have you had many different cosmetic surgery procedures at different times during your life?
___Yes ___ No

3. Are you currently under treatment or medication for anxiety or depression?
___Yes ___ No

4. Do you have a drug or alcohol problem?
___Yes ___ No

5. Are you in the middle of a life crisis?
___Yes ___ No

6. Are you preoccupied or obsessed with a part of your face or body which others do not consider unattractive?
___Yes ___ No

7. Are you suffering from depression?
___Yes ___ No
(If unsure, refer to section CD Part D for specific symptoms of depression.)

8. Are you considering cosmetic surgery primarily as a means to improve your social life, resolve marital conflicts or please someone else?
___Yes ___ No

CR Thinking It Through ЯƆ

No one consciously seeks out cosmetic surgery to worsen herself physically or psychologically, but this situation occasionally does occur. That is why, if you have answered "yes" to any of the above questions, please consider seeking out a consultation with a mental health specialist before you make this important decision for yourself. If you and your therapist both agree that cosmetic surgery would be a positive experience for you, she will be there to support you during your post surgery transition period.

You can order all ten of these *Sex, Lies and Cosmetic Surgery* printable forms in CD format at:
http://www.sexliesandcosmeticsurgery.com/
or by using the mail-in coupon at the end of this book.

CD Part D

Depression

➤ Occasional depression is not necessarily a matter of serious concern. It can be short term, provoked by a significant reality, or be a depression that does not impair your other areas of functioning.

➤ Depression as a result of bereavement, the use of a particular medication or a specific medical condition should be considered and addressed first before undergoing any elective surgery.

➤ Sometimes an adjustment to your prescribed medications or a conversation with your physician, a mental health specialist or good friend is all that is needed. It is best not to enter into elective surgery in a depressed state of mind.

➤ More deeply ingrained depressions should be recognized as such and carefully addressed. You can recognize a deeply ingrained depression if you have experienced one or more of its classic symptoms. **See ✦ note at the end of this page.**

➤ In that definition of depression, the person needs to be experiencing one or more of its specific symptoms fairly consistently during a five week period, and be feeling significant distress or impairment in social, occupational or other important areas of functioning as a result.

➤ If you think you might be experiencing depression, consider the following statements and ask yourself if any of them apply to you.

✦ Note: Listed symptoms from the Diagnostic and Statistical Manual of Mental Disorders, 4th edition, DSM-IV-TR, Published by the American Psychiatric Association, Washington, D.C. 2000, Page 356.

Signs of Depression
Which statements apply to you? ✓ Yes or No.

1. Depressed mood *most of the time nearly every day*, as indicated by either subjective report (e.g. feeling sad or empty) or observation by others (e.g. appears tearful)
_____ **Yes** _____ **No**

2. Markedly diminished interest or pleasure in all or almost all activities that previously gave you satisfaction, *most of the day, nearly every day*
_____ **Yes** _____ **No**

3. Significant weight loss when not dieting or weight gain (e.g. a change of 5 % of body weight in a month when you were not dieting)
_____ **Yes** _____ **No**

4. Decreased or increased appetite, especially in the absence of the ability to enjoy food
_____ **Yes** _____ **No**

5. Insomnia or prolonged sleep episodes *nearly every day.* (e.g. having frequent difficulty falling asleep or staying asleep, or conversely, sleeping too much)
_____ **Yes** _____ **No**

6. Body or speech agitation or retardation observable by others (e.g. restlessness, inability to sit still, pacing, hand wringing. slowed speech or body movements, speech marked by pauses, decreased volume or content)
_____ **Yes** _____ **No**

7. Fatigue or loss of energy *nearly every day*
_____ **Yes** _____ **No**

8. Feelings of worthlessness or excessive or inappropriate guilt *nearly every day* (e.g. unrealistic negative evaluation of one's self-worth or guilty preoccupation over minor past failings)
_____ **Yes** _____ **No**

9. Diminished ability to think or concentrate or indecisiveness, *nearly every day*
_____ **Yes** _____ **No**

10. Recurrent thoughts of death or suicide
_____ **Yes** _____ **No**

❧ *Thinking It through* ☙

If you have put a ✓ in front of any '*Yes*' statement(s), please seek out the services of a mental health specialist before you make the decision to undergo any elective surgery.

You can order all ten of these *Sex, Lies and Cosmetic Surgery* printable forms in CD format at:
http://www.sexliesandcosmeticsurgery.com/
or by using the mail-in coupon at the end of this book.

CD Part E

Questions to Ask *Before* You Schedule a Consultation

☙❧

Before You Schedule a Consultation

➤ You can get further accurate information about your specific list of potential surgeons via the toll free telephone numbers and Internet resources listed in Appendices 6 and 7 on Pages 326-332.

➤ Use the Internet to get answers to your Two R's, **R**eferrals (optional), and **R**eferences (mandatory), detailed in Appendix 4, Pages 318-322.

➤ Being a computer illiterate is no excuse! If you are not computer savvy, enlist the services of a reference librarian at your public library. Begin your third R, **R**esearch, by getting answers to as many of these next questions as possible.

Get Answers to These Questions Before You Schedule a Consultation:

Name of surgeon: _____

1. Is the doctor board certified by the American Board of Medical Specialties? If so, by which board or boards? **See ✤ note at the end of Part E.**

_____
_____

2. Is this a legitimate board recognized by the ABMS and does this board directly relate to your needs? (For example, you want to use a board certified Plastic Surgeon to do any surgery on your body, whereas a board certified Head and Neck Specialist might be an equally good choice for surgery to part of your face.) Remember: *Any* board certified physician is legally allowed to perform cosmetic surgery. Be cautious. **See ✤ note at the end of Part E.**

_____

3. What are this surgeon's hospital affiliations?

_____
_____

4. Does he have privileges at these hospitals to perform the surgical procedures you want?

☞ **This is critical even if your surgery is to take place in an ambulatory surgical suite.**

_____

5. Did he complete a full time cosmetic surgery fellowship? Where? For how long? _____

☞ **Look for a full time six month to one year fellowship.**

6. What percentage of his practice involves cosmetic surgery? Reconstructive surgery? _____

🗝 **Look for a surgeon whose practice has been primarily dedicated to cosmetic surgery for ten or more years.**

7. What five or six procedures does he perform most frequently? _____

🗝 **If the procedure(s) you want are <u>not</u> on his most performed list, reconsider this surgeon as one of your choices.**

8. How many of these most commonly performed procedures does he perform in a year?
_____

🗝 **Number of procedures in the range of 100 or more are desirable.**

_____
_____

9. Where does this doctor perform his surgeries? If an office or outpatient surgery facility is used, is it accredited and by whom?_____

🗝 **If not licensed by the state or accredited by AAASF, AAAHC or JCAHO, do not consider this surgeon.**

10. Who administers the anesthesia? Does he specialize in anesthesia for cosmetic surgery?

_____
_____

🗝 **You want a board certified anesthesiologist to administer your anesthesia. One who further specializes in cosmetic surgery is an additional bonus.**

11. With what other types of medically related activities has this surgeon been involved?

_____

_____

☞ **Has he authored books or journal articles on cosmetic procedures, is/was he a medical school faculty member, is he an active member of a local, state or national medical society? If so, get details.**

11. Is there a consultation fee? _____

☞ **If so, ask if this charge can be deducted from his surgical fee.**

☙❦

➤ After you have gotten answers to most if not all of these questions, place the names of your potential surgeons in a priority order list. If you have been unable to get answers to all these questions, call the first name on your list and ask to speak with their office manager. Explain that you would like to get some background information before your consultation and ask your unanswered question(s).

➤ **But please be certain you do your homework first. No office manager can spend sufficient time on one call to answer all the questions on this list, so it is essential that you do your homework to get as many answers as possible in advance of placing that call.**

➤ If you are satisfied with the answers you receive, schedule a consultation. If not, move on to the next plastic surgeon on your list. You should have at least two in-person consultations because these experiences will help sharpen your senses as to who will be right for you. On the other hand, more than three consultations might be overkill. Remember, you may be charged handsomely for each consultation, so do not treat this as a shopping expedition.

🔑 Note: If in doubt about board certification or whether his designated board is a legitimate board certified by the American Board of Medical Specialties, call: 847-491-9091 or go to: www.abms.org to check credentials.

CD Part F

Questions to Ask During Your Consultation

You come to a consultation to gain as much additional information about this surgeon as possible. Use your time while seated in his waiting room to do just that. If there is any printed material about him on display, ask for copies to take home and read at leisure. The staff at the front desk, as well as the nurse who escorts you to an examining room, will be able to provide you with additional literature about the procedures that relate to your needs.

⚕

During Your Consultation

➤ On the next four pages you will find two separate forms with groups of questions for you to ask during a consultation.

➤ The first set contains fifteen questions. Answers to these questions will give you most of the information you probably will want to know, but may not think to ask.

➤ The second set contains ten optional, additional questions. Select the ones from this list that interest you.

➤ You won't forget to ask any of these important questions if you print out copies of these forms to have on hand at your consultations.

Get Answers to These Questions During Your Consultation

Set One – Questions for the Surgeon

1. What procedures do you recommend?
☞ **Do you respond favorably to this surgeon's recommendations?**

_____

_____

2. What is your experience in performing these procedures? How many of each of these procedures have you performed in the last year? Ten years?
☞ **Remember, we all hone our skills through repetition. Look for surgical experience with a given procedure in the range of one hundred or more.**

_____

_____

3. Where will my incisions be placed?
☞ **Hold up a hand mirror so you understand specific placement of possible scars. If the placement he suggests concerns you, ask about other options.**

_____

_____

4. What are the possible risks to these procedures?
☞ **You should know that every surgery entails some risk. Know what they are.**

_____

_____

5. What is the most serious complication you have experienced from the procedures you are recommending for me?

_____

_____

6. How do you avoid those tell tale signs of surgery?

☞ **Some you want to avoid include a startled look, tight face, pale skin, lumpiness . . .**

_____

_____

7. If anesthesia will be administered, what kind will I be given?

☞ **Ask if you will be intebated or breathing on your own without the assistance of a breathing tube?**

_____

_____

8. Do you do all of the surgery yourself or does anyone assist you?

_____

_____

9. What will be the total cost of my surgery?

☞ **Does this fee include surgical facility charges, anesthesiologist's fee, recovery facility or nurse attendant, post op appointments?**

_____

_____

10. What is your policy about revision or touch up surgery, if this becomes necessary?

_____

_____

11. Do I need to hire a nurse or other professional to help me during the early stages of recovery? If so, what is your recommendation?

_____

_____

CD Part F-2

Other Questions You Might Want to Ask

Set Two – Optional Questions

Select any additional questions from the list below that seem important to you.

1. Will I experience much post-operative discomfort? If so, what do you recommend for pain control?

_____

_____

2. What do you estimate will be the expected length of time from start to finish of my surgery?

_____

_____

3. Can you prescribe some medication to help me relax before my surgery?

_____

_____

4. How many days will it take, on average, before I can leave the house? Engage in social activities? Resume my normal life style?

_____

_____

5. How long do you estimate that the beneficial effects of my surgery will last?

_____

_____

6. (If this is a relatively new technique): What training have you completed in this technique? Do you have any certificates of training in this area?

_____

_____

7. Are there alternate surgical or non-surgical techniques that you or other surgeons sometimes recommend to get similar results?

_____

_____

8. If so, what are the advantages and disadvantages of these different techniques?

_____

_____

9. Would I be able to speak with any of your patients who have had the same procedure(s)?

_____

_____

10. What attracted you to the field of plastic surgery?

_____

_____

You can order all ten of these _Sex, Lies and Cosmetic Surgery_ printable forms in CD format at:
http://www.sexliesandcosmeticsurgery.com/
or by using the mail-in coupon at the end of this book.

CD Part G

Rate Your Reaction to Your Consultation

✂

➤ Successful Cosmetic Surgery is part art and part skill. It is easier to evaluate the latter, based on the physician's training, experience and professional contributions; but you can sometimes get some idea of a surgeon's sense of artistry as well.

➤ Do his comments tell you anything about his attention to detail or does he make astute observations about your appearance? (Example: "Your right eye is more rounded, whereas your left eye is more almond shaped.") or was there anything else that impressed you about his esthetic sensibilities?

➤ This self-evaluation form lists some important criteria to consider when selecting your plastic surgeon. It is designed to help you with the third R – Personal Reaction, after each consultation.

Instructions

Rate each of the criteria that follows on a five point scale, from 5 (excellent) to 1 (poor) by circling the number that applies to your feelings about this surgeon.

Rate Your Reaction to Your Consultation

1. Do I feel a sense of integrity, competency and trust in this doctor?

Excellent   *Poor*

5   4   3   2   1

2. When I ask questions, do I understand his answers and do those answers satisfy me? **(If you didn't fully understand an answer, don't downgrade the doctor. Just rephrase the question and ask it again.)**

Excellent   *Poor*

5   4   3   2   1

3. How do I relate to him on an interpersonal level?

Excellent   *Poor*

5   4   3   2   1

4. Does he ask for and listen to my concerns?

Excellent   *Poor*

5   4   3   2   1

5. How positively do I react to the surgical recommendation(s) he has made for me?

Excellent   *Poor*

5   4   3   2   1

6. Do I leave with a feeling that this office is run in a friendly but orderly and well-structured manner?

Excellent   *Poor*

5   4   3   2   1

7. How would I rate my overall comfort level?

Excellent   *Poor*
5   4   3   2   1

8. Do I get the sense that he has artistic vision or flair?

Excellent   *Poor*
5   4   3   2   1

___**Total Score**

⚷ *How to Interpret Your Score:*

> ➤ **If your total score falls between 1 - 28:**
> You should schedule a consultation with
> the next plastic surgeon on your list.

> ➤ **If your total score falls between 29 - 35:**
> Ask yourself: "If I were given satisfactory answers
> to questions that remain in my mind, would my total
> score jump into a higher range?" If so, by all means
> first call that office and seek clarification of some of
> your questions or return to this surgeon's office for
> an additional appointment.

> ➤ **If your total score falls between 36 - 39:**
> You may have found your plastic surgeon or you
> might want to schedule a consultation with the next
> surgeon on your list, just to make sure.

> ➤ **If your total score is 40:**
> You are probably ready to sign on the dotted line.

CD Part H

Timeline Checklists ~ What to Do, When

You want to be mentally, physically and organizationally prepared for your surgery. I developed these pre-surgery timeline checklists as a result of input from plastic surgeons, cosmetic surgery nurses, estheticians and Internet resources. I then asked Cookie Levy, a highly experienced, competent cosmetic surgery RN to review them for accuracy and further insights.

You won't forget a thing if you use these timeline checklists.

❧ How to begin ❧

➤ Buy a binder or loose leaf notebook to hold all your notes, including the printable self-assessments, checklists and quizzes you choose to use from the CD forms of *Sex, Lies and Cosmetic Surgery.*

➤ Develop a mindset where you become a partner with your surgeon. Understand that if you carefully follow his advice and these checklist guidelines, you will be helping him achieve the best results for you with the fewest complications.

➤ Make an accurate and forthright list of your health history and all your health related habits to share with your surgeon. Use the form that follows to help you.

Your List:

**Forget embarrassment and go for full disclosure.
This is your life. Respect it.**

Medical conditions

_____

_____

_____

Prior Surgeries (Specify year and type)
Cosmetic surgeries _____

_____

Other surgeries _____

_____

Health Habits
Cigarettes per day _____

Amount of alcohol per day _____
(Include wine and beer.)

Use of appetite suppressants _____
                              (type/frequency)

Antidepressants _____
                              (type/frequency)

Sleeping pills or diet aids_____
                              (type/frequency)

Illicit drugs as cocaine, marijuana _____
                              (type/frequency)

_____

Medications including over the counter and prescriptive drugs and aspirin based products

_____

(type/frequency)

_____

_____

Herbal, botanical and vitamin supplements

_____

(type/frequency)

_____

☙ *Two or more <u>months</u> before surgery:* ❧

➤ If you are a smoker, try to kick the habit now. Smoking can destroy skin cells on your face. It can prevent your incisions from healing properly and possibly cause scarring. Smoking can compromise your breathing and capillary function while under anesthesia. It can also contribute to the formation of blood clots.

☛ **Do not under any circumstances try to deceive your doctor. He needs to know this information in advance, as does your anesthesiologist, who might choose to select and monitor your anesthesia differently if you are a smoker.**

➤ If you want to lose weight and are having a facelift, try to diet now.

☛ **Your face sags the most after weight loss. Let your cheeks and jowls do their sagging before surgery to help your surgeon get his best result.**

➤ If you are not staying in an overnight facility, it is highly recommended that you engage the services of a post-surgery nurse for 24-48 hours following many procedures. Ask your surgeon if this would be important for you.

➤ Educate yourself about the procedures you are scheduled to undergo.

☞ See Appendices 6 and 7, pages 326-332, for some suggested resources.

➤ Schedule your surgery to allow adequate, non-pressured time for recovery.

☞ In other words, 2 weeks before your daughter's wedding is no time to undergo cosmetic surgery.

➤ If you are having any form of facial surgery, begin to work with a knowledgeable esthetician now.

☞

The Duchess of Dermis, MICHELLE MARTEL, explains the importance of preparing your skin for facial surgery:

"If you are committed to optimal surgical results, an absolute prerequisite is good preparation of the skin, which needs to be stimulated to produce new cell growth. If your skin is well prepared to produce new collagen, has an improved texture and is rid of barnacles (those growths that appear from nowhere), hyperplasias (overactive sebacious cysts) and discolorations; the surgeon has something healthier to work with. There is more blood flow in healthier skin, which translates to healthier vascular activity.'

"If you are having any form of facial surgery, engage the services of a knowledgeable esthetician, ideally 2-3 months before surgery. When you work with a trainer, you first determine where you are now and where you want to be. Work similarly with your esthetician to develop a program for healthier skin."

➤ Avoid more than moderate use of alcohol, cigarettes, or any other drugs or products which your doctor has cautioned you against.

☞ **If you need to detoxify from more than moderate use of alcohol, nicotine, recreational drugs, blood thinning medications and more, speak to your surgeon and elicit his assistance.**

➤ Avoid crash diets.

➤ Clear your calendar of all work, social and family obligations for a minimum of two weeks beyond your date of surgery unless your surgeon advises you differently.

☞ **Pretend you are going on a vacation to Hawaii and block out this vacation time on your calendar with no commitments to anyone except yourself.**

➤ Schedule your pre-op appointment with your internist.

➤ Arrange to have a spouse, parent or friend home with you for an additional 24 hours after the first 24 hours of nursing care, unless you have engaged a nurse for additional hours.

CR *Two weeks before surgery* SO

➤ For shop-at-home convenience, if you want to order specialty items specifically designed for recovery after various surgical procedures, check out Home Recovery's online catalogue at: http://www.homerecovery.com/.

☞ **These folks have thought about absolutely everything: e.g. floppy hat with attached scarf, pillow with proper head elevation after a facelift, special undergarments to wear after body surgery; and their items are well priced. But you need to order now to avoid last minute hassles.**

➤ Continue to avoid all of the ingredients listed earlier plus any aspirin based medications, non-steroidal or anti-inflammatory medications, diuretics and the vitamins, herbs, foods and other remedies your doctor has instructed you to avoid at this time.

➤ If you still are a smoker, stop <u>all</u> smoking now. If you consume alcohol or use any recreational drugs, <u>completely</u> discontinue their use now.

➤ Avoid people who are likely to fill you with negative thoughts. Instead, surround yourself with a nucleus of people who will support and encourage you.
☞ **It has been shown that people who go into surgery feeling confident and positive about their surgical outcome generally have fewer complications and heal more quickly.**

➤ If you are the jittery type, select and continue to practice one of the relaxation techniques described in Appendix 5, Pages 323-325.
☞ **If you want some medication to help you relax, ask your doctor for a prescription, but <u>do</u> <u>not</u> take any medication without his approval.**

➤ Give yourself a mental mindset of a minimum of two weeks for healing.

ೞ *The week before surgery* ೞ

➤ Gather together the items needed or recommended for your post surgery care.

☛ **If you have not been given a list, request one.**

➤ Fill any prescriptions given to you by your surgeon.

➤ Purchase stool softener if your surgeon has prescribed painkillers.

➤ Purchase the foods you will need for the first few days after surgery. Avoid spicy foods after any type surgery.

☛ **If a soft diet is recommended, blended nutritional soups, protein shakes blended with berries or bananas, applesauce, Oysterettes, yogurts and cottage cheese work well.**

➤ Stock your freezer with lots of ice. Frozen peas in zip lock bags make great facial cold packs.

➤ Think through your desire for confidentiality and disclosure. Decide whom you will tell and how much.

☛ **For those you do not plan to tell, prepare and rehearse an explanation for your enhanced appearance in advance so that your words sound believable.**

ೞ *Optional ideas* ೞ

➤ It's a real bonus to have a responsible adult available to help with necessary tasks or to just keep you company while you continue to recuperate after nursing care is no longer needed. Try to arrange this in advance.

➤ Have someone take some pre-surgery close up photos of you, which reveal your facial features or body contours scheduled for enhancement.

☞ **Although your surgeon will take photographs for his records, it's helpful to have some of your own for future reference. It's amazing how quickly you are likely to forget the appearance of the former you.**

➤ Borrow book tapes, CD's or videos from your local library.

➤ Purchase or borrow a speakerphone if you are having facial surgery.

➤ Obtain crossword puzzle books, magazines or other light reading material.

➤ Get your hair cut or restyled and freshly colored.

➤ Have a relaxing body massage or aromatherapy session.

Denise Thomas recommends Optimal Outcome Skincare Products for rapid healing of the skin after any cosmetic surgical procedure.

❦ *The day before surgery* ❧

➤ Arrange your recovery space.
☞ **Pillows, towels, fresh sleepwear, small ice chest, gauze pads, toiletries and medications**

➤ Place all prescription medications, including those you normally take and those prescribed by your surgeon, on a table in your recovery room, along with a chart or written instructions of what to take when.
☞ **Snack size zip lock bags work well if you label them carefully by date and approximate time to be taken.**

☛ **If a particular medication needs to be taken in a specific way as:** *"Take on an empty stomach", "Take with food"* **or** *"Take with a full glass of water"*, **you need to place that medication in a separate zip lock bag and include those instructions on the label.**

➤ Gather together all the recommended toiletries.

☛ **Some helpful items to have on hand might include gentle shampoo and a lotion cleanser, mouthwash, Q-tips, child size toothbrush, gentle body wash**

➤ Focus on the positives of the new you - how wonderful you will look and feel after your recovery.

➤ Calm your mind.

☛ **Remember to focus on the competence of your surgeon and to use the relaxation techniques described in Appendix 5.**

➤ Do not eat any food or drink any liquids after midnight before the day of your scheduled surgery.

☛ **Do not cheat here. While anesthetized, a person loses the ability to cough up gastric contents, if they should be inhaled. These instructions are for your benefit and safety.**

○ੴ *The day of surgery* ☙

➤ Read over the day of surgery instructions your doctor has given you.

➤ Do at least one of the relaxation exercise from Appendix 5, Pages 323-325.

➤ Keep your mind focused on:

☛ **The competence of your surgeon**

☛ **The excitement of discovering the new you and the transformation you are about to experience.**

CD Part I

Test Your Body Image

Instructions

This printable checklist has ten statements pertaining to body image. Using the seven point value scale below, write a number on the line in front of each statement to indicate how strongly it relates to your feelings about your physical appearance.

7: Strongly agree
6: Mostly agree
5: Slightly agree
4: Neither agree nor disagree
3: Slightly disagree
2: Mostly disagree
1: Strongly disagree.

_____ **1.** Most people would consider me attractive.

_____ **2.** I think I have an attractive face.

_____ **3.** When I get undressed, I like the reflection that I see in the mirror.

_____ **4.** I think my body is physically attractive.

_____ **5.** I like the way I look when I get dressed in clothes.

_____ **6.** I think my body is sexually appealing.

_____ **7.** When I put on make-up and fix my hair, I generally like the reflection I see in the mirror.

_____ **8.** I feel feminine and sexually attractive.

_____ **9.** When I go out, I generally feel good about my physical appearance.

_____ **10.** I think of my physically appearance as an asset when I meet new people.

_____**Total Score**

How to Interpret Your Score:

Total Score range 70 - 65: Very strong body image

Total Score range 64 – 59 Good body image

Total Score range 58 – 45 Average body image

Total Score range 44 – 35 Below average body image

Total Score range 34 or below: Poor body image

You can order all ten of these *Sex, Lies and Cosmetic Surgery* printable forms in CD format at:
http://www.sexliesandcosmeticsurgery.com/
or by using the mail-in coupon at the end of this book.

CD Part J

Body Dysmorphic Disorder Checklist (BDD)

Incidences of BDD are increasing in the USA, due to media and attitudinal changes in our society. This printable checklist will help you answer the question:

"Is it possible that I am suffering from BDD?"

Instructions

Put a ✓ in front of *Yes* or *No to* answer each question.

1. Are you dissatisfied with your overall body image rather than a specific feature of your appearance?
___ **Yes** ___ **No**

2. Does your dissatisfaction preoccupy your thoughts and/or result in time consuming behaviors for at least one hour per day? ___ **Yes** ___ **No**

3. If you are preoccupied with thoughts or actions about your appearance, do these thoughts or actions impair you from participating in other activities or result in non-attendance at social events, at work, at school, etc.?
___ **Yes** ___ **No**

4. Are you dissatisfied or preoccupied with a defect that others do not recognize or that others consider quite minor? ___ **Yes** ___ **No**

5. Do you repeatedly check or examine yourself or avoid social contacts because of your poor body image?
___ **Yes** ___ **No**

6. Have you tried to correct this defect through repeated cosmetic surgeries or other medical treatments that have proven ineffective? ___ **Yes** ___ **No**

7. Do you pick at your skin, some part of your face or nose? ___ **Yes** ___ **No**

8. Do you find it difficult to meet new people or make new friends because of concerns that your appearance will be judged negatively? ___ **Yes** ___ **No**

How to Interpret Your Score:

If you answered *Yes* to any of these questions, please consider the following points below:

▶ No one consciously seeks out cosmetic surgery to worsen herself physically or psychologically, but this situation does occasionally occur. That is why, if you have answered "yes" to any of the above statements, please consider seeking out a consultation with a professional therapist with a good understanding of body image constructs before you make this important decision for yourself.

▶ Research suggests that some people who have BDD still benefit from cosmetic surgery, but in other cases their symptoms worsen when surgery does not bring about the hoped for psychological changes. This is an unfortunate result for patient and surgeon alike.

▶ If you and your therapist both agree that cosmetic surgery would be a positive experience for you at this time, you will have established a built in support system in advance to use during your post surgery transition period, if you feel the need.

$$\mathscr{Appendices}$$

	Page
Appendix 1: Meet Denise Thomas	301
Appendix 2: Anatomy of an Interview (How I structured my interviews)	305
Appendix 3: My Cosmetic Surgery Questionnaire	307
Appendix 4: Selecting Your Surgeon – The First Two R's	318
Appendix 5: Relaxation Techniques – Ways to Calm Your Mind	323
Appendix 6: Internet and Book Resources	326
Appendix 7: Associations, Medical Boards, Web-sites and More	331
Appendix 8: Personal Profiles	333
Appendix 9: Additional Stories	364

Appendix 1: Meet Denise Thomas

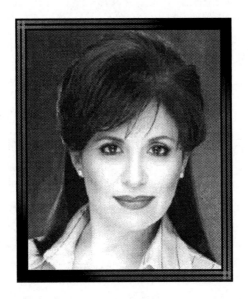

Denise, New York's Cosmetic Surgery Consultant, has a keen eye for matching each of her clients with just the right Board Certified plastic surgeon to meet their surgical needs. This also applies to cosmetic dentists and dermatologists. If clients want further input, she is happy to oblige. Denise is a most attractive brunette with a professional, refined manner. She uses her twenty-seven years of experience and her insider connections to hone her ability to differentiate between highly credentialed surgeons and those simply with good P.R.

How Denise Goes About Her Work

After a client contacts Denise, they usually meet in her Upper East Side office to explore individual needs. Denise matches each client with a plastic surgeon skilled in those particular areas. She explains:

> "Some plastic surgeon have more expertise with faces than body work, and consequently may not get the best results with breasts or necks. Others do fantastic noses. Some are just plain good at everything. "That's where I come in. It's important for me to get the right match between the needs of my client and the doctor's particular skills. Some of my clients have specific budgetary or doctor personality needs as well. I am sensitive to all these factors and take them into consideration before making final recommendations. After all, that is what I am being paid to do."

Many people choose to use Denise's services because she is able to facilitate the entire process. She works to increase each client's comfort level by sharing relevant information with the office staff before any of her clients enter the physician's office. "My clients tell me that from the moment they walk in the door, they feel welcome and at ease. That's such a reassuring feeling for someone about to undertake any surgical procedure."

I asked Denise how she goes about the important process of selecting the surgeons she recommends. Here is what she explained about her criteria.

"I'm extremely strict. First, they must be Board Certified plastic surgeons. I won't even consider a surgeon who is not Board Certified in plastic surgery. I need to see their work for at least two years before I will recommend them. I look at their education. I want the doctors who have received the best education, the Ivy Leaguers or those from similar caliber schools. I've been a consultant for over twenty-seven years, so I've culled quite a strong list from my years of experience. I get input on plastic surgeons from anesthesiologists, nurses and former patients. They can be surprisingly on target in their assessment of the work of various plastic surgeons. They see the results daily."

How People Learn About Denise

Denise has appeared as a guest on a number of TV shows including Oprah, Fox News Channel and Discovery Channel, to name a few. Exposure from those shows has made people more aware of what she actually does, how she can best help. Her attractive bi-monthly ad in New York magazine heightens awareness for others. And of course she gets lots of referrals from happy clients, their friends and even their spouses.

When prospective clients contact Denise, if possible, they meet with her in her office. If a client is too busy or lives out of state, as her West Coast and Southern clients, e-mailing her their photos suffices. High profile personalities who require total anonymity will send a car to deliver Denise to a private destination to avoid being spotted entering her office.

Denise does all the leg work and research to make sure the right doctors are available to her clients when they need them and imparts invaluable information to them.

Denise concludes:

> "When you go to my website, you will see the words:
> *Youth and Beauty are Power Tools.* I really believe
> that's the bottom line. It's such an asset when you are
> in the business world to look younger and more
> attractive. People generally prefer to associate with
> people who look more appealing. Also, you project a
> more exuberant attitude when you look and feel your
> best. So cosmetic surgery, with the right doctor of
> course, works on two levels: it enhances the
> individual's appearance and personality as well."

I told Denise that my Dad used to preach: *Do something that
you absolutely love and you will be successful at it.* He was
right. Denise's enthusiasm and sense of fulfillment in her
work epitomizes my Dad's philosophy of success.

Appendix 2: The Anatomy of an Interview

Structuring My Personal Interviews

I began this book as a personal journal, my private journey into the world of cosmetic surgery, but as I began to create my manuscript, I decided to blend my experiences with those of other women. To that end, I developed a questionnaire for women who had undergone cosmetic surgery, posted it on a private Internet site and invited women to respond anonymously.

As an introduction to the section of my questionnaire relating to sexual activity, I advised respondents who were not sexually active to simply skip those questions and move on to the next section. Some expressed a sense of renewal after surgery. Others agreed that they felt more sensual, but said no more. Still others said that nothing had changed for them or skipped that set of questions and continued on to safer ground. I was left to ponder the possibilities. Perhaps they were afraid I would track them, discover their identities and misuse the information. Perhaps they considered my questions too personal or even irrelevant. A woman who identified herself by the code name **'Jockette'** wrote: *I didn't see the need for some of these questions. They made me feel uncomfortable and wonder if that is just me or if others felt similarly.* Answers to other questions were similarly cryptic and sparse. I wasn't getting the open-ended discussion I was seeking.

Eventually I abandoned the questionnaire format in favor of personal interviews, most times conducted by phone, but I used questions from my questionnaire as a basis for these conversations. I networked through clinical estheticians, cosmetic surgery nurses, personal trainers, Internet support groups, friends and acquaintances and Denise Thomas, the Cosmetic Surgery Consultant whose thoughts are found within many chapters of this book. I made fliers for distribution at upscale gyms and posted notices in select publications, inviting women to participate in confidential interviews. Through these varied venues, I was able to listen to the voices of over one hundred women. Their honesty and candor added considerable insight to many of my chapters.

During each interview I worked to increase the respondent's comfort level by building rapport. I gave them the following assurances: **a)** Any information we shared would be kept totally confidential. **b)** Only first names, or fictitious names if they preferred, would be used for identification purposes. **c)** We would maintain an open forum, which meant that they could ask me questions as well as answer those I asked of them. **d)** They would have editing rights. I would give them an opportunity to read and approve or edit the contents pertaining to our interview prior to publication. **e)** They had the right to remain silent or tell me they preferred to skip a particular question. Furthermore, if I sensed that someone was clearly uncomfortable with a topic, I simply moved on.

Conducting these interviews was a rewarding experience for me. I met such a wide range of interesting women and became further enlightened with each of our conversations. Some of them have become my extended family of friends, a further blessing I received as a result of writing this book.

CR

Appendix 3 - My Cosmetic Surgery Questionnaire

Kindly print all your responses.

CODE NAME: Please record the name or pseudonym you would like to use in the event that some of your written comments are selected for publication.

IMPORTANT: Record your code name here.

_____

I am particularly interested in personal stories relevant to your cosmetic surgery experience, especially those which present amusing anecdotes, fresh insights, confidences, interesting viewpoints and/or dramatic moments.

**Worried about revealing your identity? You can open a FREE e-mail account with a pseudonym of your choice at: http://www.mail@yahoo.com/

PART ONE - BEFORE SURGERY:

1. What particular events propelled you toward cosmetic surgery?
(Please put 1 next to all events which were most significant for you, 2 next to events of moderate significance and 3 next to those of lesser significance. Place a 0 next to any statement that does not apply.)

a) ___ Being unnerved by a particular photograph or mirror image of myself

b) ___ Seeing positive cosmetic surgery results obtained by someone else

c) ___ Being mistaken for older than my actual age

d) ___ Hearing a hurtful comment about my physical appearance

e) ___ Low self-esteem

f) ___ Self-consciousness about a specific feature of my face or body

g) ___ Desire to improve social aspects of my life

h) ___ Medical necessity

i) ___

Other_____

2. Please tell the story or specifics about at least one of the events you numbered 1 or 2 above. (Please PRINT or TYPE.)

3. Tell about any ambivalent feelings you experienced when you began to think in terms of cosmetic surgery. (i.e. feeling that you were being: self-indulgent, vain, looking for trouble, should be using your money differently, etc.) **(Please PRINT or TYPE.)**

4. Tell about the emotions you experienced prior to surgery. (i.e. excited, proud, embarrassed, fearful, etc.) **(Please PRINT or TYPE.)**

5. Please indicate the criteria you consider most important in selecting a plastic surgeon? (Please put 1 next to all criteria you consider most important, 2 next to those of moderate importance and 3 next to criteria of lesser importance to you. Place 0 next to any statement that you think is unimportant.)

a) ___ Quality of doctor's formal education and training
b) ___ Keeping up to date on newest techniques through continuing education
c) ___ Artistically talented
d) ___ Responsive to patient's expressed needs and concerns
e) ___ Active, involved member of the ASAPS (American Society for Aesthetic Plastic Surgery)
f) ___ Certified at affiliated hospitals to perform the specific procedures you need
g) ___ Number of years of experience
h) ___ Other_____

6. How did you select your plastic surgeon? (Please put 1 next to all statements which influenced you most strongly, 2 next to those of moderate influence, 3 next to those of minimal influence. Put 0 if statement did not apply to you.)

a) ____ Recommended by a friend who had used this surgeon.
b) ____ Word of mouth recommendation
c) ____ Recommended by another physician
d) ____ Recommended by a cosmetic surgery consultant
e)____ Contacted hospital or professional organization as the ASAPS (American Society for Aesthetic Plastic Surgery) for a recommendation.
f) ____ Internet search
g)____ Other

7. Rate your level of self-consciousness about your appearance prior to your surgery? On a scale of 1 to 5, let 1 represent extreme self-consciousness and 5 represent minimal self-consciousness.

_____ = Your self-consciousness rating sale

If you felt self-conscious, please detail the areas of your face or body that caused those feelings.

8. On a scale of 1- 5, how would you have rated your appearance *prior to* cosmetic surgery? (Let 1 represent below average attractiveness AND 5 represent extremely attractive.)

_____ = Your prior-to-surgery personal appearance rating

9. Using this same 1-5 scale, how do you think others would have rated you?

_____ = Your prior-to-surgery appearance rating as assessed by others

10. What were your personal motivations for cosmetic surgery?
(Please put 1 next to your strongest reasons, 2 next to your reasons of moderate importance and 3 for reasons that were less significant to you yet still applied. Put 0 next to any statement that did not apply to you.)

a)___ Preserve my youthful appearance
b)___ Rectify what nature did not provide
c)___ Attract new partners
d)___ Improve my perceptions, thoughts and feelings about myself
e)___ Correct a medical condition
f)___ Help me look as young as I feel
g)___ Other _____

11. Please tell your own story of any specific event, conversation, observation, etc. which encouraged you to have cosmetic surgery.
(i.e. reflection in mirror, hurtful comment, a photograph, feeling ignored or rejected, etc.) **(Please PRINT or TYPE.)**

12. Pretend that you are standing on a ladder where the 1st rung represents the worst possible life and the 10th rung represents the ideal, happiest life. Which rung would you have been standing on the year before your surgery?

_____ = Your pre-surgery happiness rating

13. Please put the date of each surgery (mm/yyyy) next to any cosmetic procedure you have ever had at any time in your life.

a) _____ Eyelid tightening (Blepharoplasty)

309

b) _____ Breast augmentation
c) _____ Breast reduction
d) _____ Face lift (Rhytidectomy)
e) _____ Liposuction
f) _____ Tummy tuck (Abdominoplasty)
g) _____ Chin implant (Genioplasty)
h) _____ Forehead lift
i) _____ Nose reshaping (Rhinoplasty)
j) _____ Other
k) If you selected 'Other' directly above, please specify.

_____

l) If you selected liposuction above, please detail areas of body.

_____

14. Please put an (X) next to the statement that best reflects your feelings about financing your cosmetic surgery?

a) ____ Payment was easy and required no lifestyle changes.
b) ____ Payment took some sacrifices (as giving up a special vacation), but had no other impact.
c) ____ Payment took great sacrifice (as taking an additional part time job or loan), but was worth every penny.
d) ____ Payment took great sacrifice and I regret this expense.
e) ____ Other_____

15. Why do you think some people might avoid cosmetic surgery?
(Please put 1 next to the statements you think might be the strongest reasons, 2 for reasons of moderate importance and 3 for reasons of lesser importance. Put 0 next to any statement that you consider irrelevant.)

a) ____ Fear of pain
b) ____ Fear of permanent damage
c) ____ Appearance is not a high priority to them
d) ____ Concern about a lengthy recovery
e) ____ Financial concerns
f) ____ Goes against personal beliefs
g) ____ Fear of anesthesia
h) ____ Other _____

16. Please explain the statements you rated 1 or 2 above.

17. Why do you think many people maintain an aura of secrecy about their cosmetic surgery? (Please PRINT or TYPE.)

18. Please tell your story of your feelings of calm or jitteriness prior to your cosmetic surgery. Did you do anything special to calm yourself? (Please PRINT or TYPE.)

PART TWO - AFTER SURGERY:

19. On a scale of 1-5, with <u>1 being the lowest and 5 being the highest</u>, please rate your level of overall satisfaction with the results of your cosmetic surgery.

_____ = Your satisfaction rating

20. How would you compare your post surgery physical appearance with your appearance prior to surgery? (i.e. dramatic improvement, much improved, moderate improvement, somewhat improved, slight improvement, worse than before).

21. Please describe your recovery following cosmetic surgery in terms of healing time and amount of discomfort you experienced. (i.e. healed faster/slower than I anticipated, experienced a minimum/more discomfort than anticipated, etc.).

22. How many days did it take before you felt sufficiently healed to go out in public?
a) _____ days
How many days did it take before you felt sufficiently healed to attend social functions?
b) _____ days

23. Which statements relate to personal changes you have made, if any, since your cosmetic surgery? (Please put 1 next to your most obvious changes, 2 next to moderate changes and 3 for the most subtle changes you have made. Put 0 next to any statement that does not apply.)

a) ___ Change of hair style
b) ___ Weight loss
c) ___ More interest in skin care
d) ___ More use of cosmetics
e) ___ More use of skin care products
f) ___ Services of another professional (i.e. esthetician, body trainer)
g) ___ Look in mirror more frequently
h) ___ Heightened interest in and/or change in style of dress
i) ___ Began body exercise program
j) ___ Began facial exercises program
k) ___ Other _____

24. Which statements relate to how you feel about yourself since your cosmetic surgery? (Please put 1 next to your strongest feelings, 2 next to moderate feelings and 3 next to more subtle feelings. Put 0 next to any statement that does not apply to you.)

a) ___ Younger, more energetic
b) ___ More outgoing, friendlier
c) ___ Happier, more content
d) ___ Prettier
e) ___ More self confidant
f) ___ More sensual
g) ___ More flirtatious
h) ___ Feel the same as before
i) ___ Less friendly and less outgoing
j) ___ Less happy, less content
k)___ Less attractive
l) ___ Less sensual or less flirtatious
m) ___ Other changes _____

25. Please give some details or examples of specific episodes where you experienced any of the feelings you rated 1 or 2 above.

26. Which personal lifestyle change statements do you attribute at least in part to your cosmetic surgery? (Please put 1 next to the statements that you believe relate most strongly, 2 next to those that relate moderately and 3 next to those that relate minimally. Put 0 next to any statement that you think does not apply to you.)

a) ___ Better job or new career
b) ___ Promotion in job
c) ___ Deeper involvement in either your work or a special interest pursuit
d) ___ More participation in social activities
e) ___ Take more initiatives in social and/or job related situations
f) ___ Express opinions more openly or assertively
g) ___ More sexually active
h) ___ Less inhibited
i) ___ Less involvement in either your work or a special interest pursuit
j) ___ Less participation in social activities
k) ___ Take fewer initiatives in social and/or job related situations
l) ___ Express opinions less openly or assertively.
m) ___ Less sexually active
n) ___ More inhibited
o) ___ Other _____

27. Please give some details or specific examples of any lifestyle changes you rated 1 or 2 in question 26.

28. Pretend that you are standing on a ladder where the 1st rung represents the worst possible life and the 10th rung represents the ideal, happiest life. Which rung would you be standing on within two years after your surgery?

_____ = Your post-surgery happiness rating

29. Which statements best describe your responses toward other people since your cosmetic surgery. (Please put 1 next to your strongest responses, 2 next to your moderate responses and 3 next to minimal responses. Put 0 next to any statement that does not apply.)

a) ___ I tend to be more candid and revealing in my conversations.
b) ___ I display more humor in everyday interactions.
c) ___ I show more affection in general.
d) ___ I radiate more energy and zest for living.
e) ___ No changes noted
f) ___ I tend to be less candid and revealing in my conversations.
g) ___ I display less humor in everyday interactions.
h) ___ I show less affection in general.
i) ___ I radiate less energy and zest for living.
j) Other _____

30. Describe your early (first three months) emotional reactions following cosmetic surgery. (i.e. I felt: elated, guilty, energized, embarrassed, proud, sensual, etc.) Please give specific examples of how you manifested those emotions. (Please type or print.)

31. Please tell your story of your first post surgery look in the mirror and any memories or thoughts it evoked. (Please type or print.)

32. What differences, if any, do you notice in the way men or women respond to you since your cosmetic surgery? (Please put 1M, 1W or 1MW next to the strongest reactions you have observed from M (men) W (women) or MW (men and women), 2M, 2W or 2MW for moderate reactions and 3M, 3W or 3MW for less obvious reactions. Put a 0 next to any statement that does not apply.)

a)___ More people smile at me.

313

b)___ I receive more admiring glances.
c)___ People initiate more conversation(s) with me.
d)___ People make more physical contact with me (i.e. hugs, touching).
e)___ I am the subject of more banter and friendly teasing.
f)___ I have received more expressions of resentment.
g)___ I have felt some jealousy directed toward me.
h)___ I have sensed some disapproval.
i)___ I have noted some preferential treatment toward me. (i.e. social, business, medical, legal, etc.)
j)___ Other _____

33. Please give specific examples of either men or women's reactions that you rated 1 or 2 above.

34. On a scale of 1 to 5 (with 1 indicating minimal impact and 5 indicating greatest impact), how much do you think your post surgery physical appearance impacted upon your self-esteem?

_____ = Self-esteem rating

35. If you rated the impact on your self-esteem as 3 or higher, please give examples or tell a story of how you have exhibited this increased self-esteem.

36. In general what factors do you think contribute to your feelings of positive self-image? (Please put 1 next to the factor(s) that affect you most strongly, 2 next to factors of moderate impact and 3 next to those of minimal impact. Put 0 next to any statement that does not apply.)

a)____ Confidence in my abilities
b)____ Good relationships with family members and friends
c)____ Feeling productive
d)____ Being physically active
e)____ Being intellectually active
f)____ Experiencing feelings of accomplishment and achievement
g)____ Love from another person
h)____ My physical appearance
j)____ Having a close relationship with a spouse or significant other
k)____ Positive sexual experiences
l)____ Feeling that I am liked by others
m)____ Feeling that others enjoy my companionship
n)____Other_____

37. Please note that it is neither unusual nor abnormal to feel a special attraction toward your plastic surgeon, so try to be candid as

you assess the following statements. (Please put 1 next to your strongest responses, 2 next to moderate responses and 3 next to minimal responses. Put a 0 next to any statement that does not apply to you.)

a)___ I maintained a purely professional, non-emotional relationship with my plastic surgeon.

b)___ I felt warmed by how much he cared about me as a human being - not just as a patient.

c)___ I wondered and secretly hoped he regarded me as his favorite patient.

d)___ When I saw other clients waiting in the reception area, I wondered if he showed them as much interest.

e)___ I found my plastic surgeon increasingly attractive with each visit.

f)___ I would take great care to dress extra attractively for appointments with my plastic surgeon.

h)___ I felt unsettled by some of the feelings I was experiencing toward my plastic surgeon.

i)___ I enjoyed the sensual feelings I experienced toward my plastic surgeon.

j)___ Other _____

38. Please give examples or tell your own story about any statement you rated 1 or 2 above.

39. On a scale of 1- 5, how would you rate your appearance *following* cosmetic surgery? (Let 1 represent below average attractiveness and 5 represent extremely attractive.)

_____ = Your post surgery personal appearance rating

40. Using this same 1-5 scale, how do you think others would rate you?

_____ = Your post surgery appearance rating as assessed by others

41. Has cosmetic surgery impacted upon you as a sexual human being? (Please put 1 next to your strongest response(s), 2 next to your moderate responses and 3 next to minimal responses. Put a 0 next to any statement that does not apply to you.)

Note: If you are not sexually active, simply skip this question.

a)___ I derive more pleasure and enjoyment from sex.

b)___ I think of myself as a better sex partner.

c)___ I rate my sexual skills higher now than before my plastic surgery.

d)___ I initiate sexual encounters more frequently now than prior to surgery.

e)___ Same as before.

f)___ I derive less pleasure and enjoyment from sex.

g)___ I think of myself as a less effective sex partner.

h)___ I initiate sexual encounters less frequently now than prior to surgery.

i)___ Other_____

42. Please give examples or tell your own story about any statement you rated 1 or 2 above.

43. If you had a magic wand and could change any one thing about your face or body, what would you choose to change?

PART THREE: FACTS ABOUT YOU

44. What is your current age? _____

45. Please (X) the word that best describes your primary residence?
a)___ Urban
b)___ Suburban
c)___ Small town
d)___ Rural
e)___ Other _____

46. Please tell about your family. Do you have any children or grandchildren? If so, how many of each? (Pets are adorable, but should not be included here!)

47. How would you describe yourself? (Please put 1 next to the statements that best describe you, 2 next to statements that describe you to a moderate degree, and 3 next to those statements that describe you slightly. Put 0 next to any statement that you think does not apply to you.)

a)____ Family oriented
b)____ Relationship oriented
c)____ Career oriented
d)____ Outgoing, extroverted
e)____ Quiet, more introverted
f)____ Happy, cheerful
g)____ Worried or depressed
h)____ Spiritually oriented
i)____ Traditional values and thoughts
j)____ Liberal values and thoughts
k)____ Innovative, creative

l)____ Intellectual
m)____ Fun loving
n)____ Emotional
o)____ Rational
p)____ Serious minded
q)____ Deliberate thinker
r)____ Organized, systematic
s)____ Other _____

48. Please describe your marital status: (i.e. single, married, divorced separated, same sex partner, opposite sex partner, widowed, etc.)

49. Please list your special interest(s) and/or hobbies.

50. Please (X) the statement that best describes your level of formal education.
a)___ Completed grades 6-9
b ___ High School graduate
c)___ Completed a two year college program
d)___ College graduate
e)___ Post graduate degree(s)
f)___ Other_____

51. What do you consider your most important achievement(s) or goal(s):

52. Which statement best describes your annual household income?
a) ___ Under $50,000
b) ___ $50,000 - $99,000
c) ___ $100,000 - $150,000
d) ___ $150,000 - $200,000
e) ___ Over $200,000

Thank you ever so much for participating in this study. Your efforts are deeply appreciated.

Lois W. Stern

CR

Appendix 4: Selecting Your Surgeon
The First Two R's

There is an intelligent approach to selecting the surgeon who is right for you. I call this method:

The 3 R's - Referrals, Research and Personal Response

The First R – Referrals

➤ **You can begin your search by consulting others who might be 'in the know' and who generally make judgments you respect.** Operating Room nurses are an incredibly reliable source of accurate information. I was fortunate to have such a competent RN living next door to me, but if you don't know one personally, don't despair. You can speak with a surgery department nurse at a respected hospital in your area and ask for her valued opinion. Whom would she select for herself or a family member? (It is best to do this in person, not on the phone.)

➤ **You can sometimes receive a wealth of information from other forms of networking.** Ask a trusted physician, a friend, even your hairdresser or esthetician. These word-of-mouth recommendations may be helpful, even right on target, or totally off base; but they are one way to begin.

➤ **Many women choose a plastic surgeon based on a friend's recommendation, an advertisement or a media appearance.** In my case my plastic surgeon's name bounced back at me from multiple sources. If you know several people who have been pleased with a specific surgeon, and you like the results he has achieved, you have some good beginning references. Seek the advice of knowledgeable people whose opinions you respect, as their recommendations can often lead you to highly credentialed, skilled surgeons. But not always.

☞ Keep in mind the caveats to referrals. Be aware that referrals can be right on target or flawed advice.

☞ A fine internist may have limited knowledge of the field of plastic surgery or may routinely restrict her recommendations to specialists within her affiliated medical group.

☞ The judgments offered by friends are normally formed from a small sampling of patients, and might not accurately reflect this surgeon's expertise. Your hairstylist or cosmetician may recommend a plastic surgeon simply because she has read about him in a popular magazine or because his wife is one of her favorite clients.

☞ A name might currently be in vogue because of a recent media blitz arranged by this plastic surgeon's publicity agent, and have little to do with the doctor's skills. Referrals can be right on target or flawed advice. They are one way to begin, but your search should not end here.

The Second R – Research

➤ **The second R, Research, is a step you should never omit.** Your research is your black and white data about any plastic surgeon's training, skill and standing amongst colleagues. The Internet is a most valued resource.

☞ Being a computer illiterate is not a good excuse! Enlist the services of a reference librarian at your local library if you're not computer savvy.

➤ **Most surgeons now have their own websites,** which often provide important background information, and sometimes reflect the surgeon's personality and values as well.

☞ Be sure to also do a google-search of each prospective surgeon to see if any additional information about him is posted on the web. Print out all the information you find pertaining to this surgeon. It will help you get answers to many of your research questions.

☞ See Part E of the *Sex, Lies and Cosmetic Surgery* CD, reproduced on Pages 275-278, for a list of the questions you need to get answered *before* you schedule a consultation with any particular surgeon

➤ **But first, please read the contents of the two hypothetical websites I have created**, along with some explanatory notes, to help you read between the lines of the websites you explore:

◊◊ *Website A* ◊◊

Dr. A has achieved international recognition as a board certified plastic surgery. His textbook, Achieving the Cosmetic Surgery Results Every Patient Deserves, published in 2006, received glowing reviews in several medical journals including the New England Journal of Medicine and the Journal of Plastic and Reconstructive Surgery. Dr. A subsequently earned the James Barrett Brown Award, one of the most prestigious awards given by one's medical peers.

A notable author, lecturer, and teacher, Dr. A is an Associate Professor of Plastic Surgery at Yale Medical School and has published articles on a wide array of topics, including: Hand Rejuvenation: A New Focus in Cosmetic Surgery, in a number of well respected medical journals. An active member and past-president of the American Society for Aesthetic Plastic Surgery, he is a popular presenter at their annual conferences.

Dr. A graduated Magna Cum Laude from Harvard University where he had a dual major in fine arts and science. He served as a fellow in Plastic Surgery at New York-Presbyterian Hospital under the esteemed surgery team of . . .

Comments about the Website of Dr. A: **Every word speaks to expertise, outstanding training and respected recognition amongst peers. This surgeon's dual major at Harvard University included both science and fine arts, suggesting not just high intelligence but artistic vision as well. This is a man who selected the field of plastic surgery to embrace his special talents and has dedicated his practice to cosmetic plastic surgery (as opposed to reconstructive plastic surgery).**

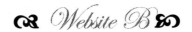
Website B

Dr. B is board certified in facial plastic surgery and has been featured in The New York Times, Elle, Vogue and many other national television and print media. Dr. B is a nationally recognized expert in cosmetic surgery. He lectures extensively on the hottest and newest cosmetic surgery techniques and is active in the teaching of students and residents at many hospitals and medical centers..

(Note: This first paragraph is superimposed over the **nude silhouette of a seductively posed, slender, curvaceous woman.**)

Dr. B believes in using the most modern techniques in attempting to make every patient as "perfect as possible" and sponsors annual fashion parades, where you can speak with his well satisfied patients and observe their beautiful surgical results.

<u>Comments about the Website of Dr. B:</u> The American Board of Medical Specialties does not list the board name with which Dr. B accredits himself. (There is no American Board of <u>Facial</u> Plastic Surgery recognized by the ABMS.) We never learn where Dr. B lectures or teaches, what he considers the "newest" techniques and how he has studied or implemented these techniques into his practice. Furthermore, his stated objective: "to make each patient as perfect as possible" is objectionable. It is honorable to strive for the best possible results, but striving to make each patient look "perfect" sounds too much like one of the Steppford Wives! It is very unlikely that Dr. B. would be accepted as a member of the ASAPS, a highly esteemed organization that disparages such forms of self-promotion.

Keep in mind that, unlike the peer reviewed professional journal articles noted on <u>Website A</u>, articles printed in popular magazines are rarely scholarly, and may be more a tribute to a surgeon's business acumen (e.g. his ability to garner publicity and increase magazine sales) than to his professional expertise. I objected to his choice of jargon. "Hottest" is fine when it comes to fashion, but when it comes to cosmetic surgery, I want my face to look refreshed and natural, not trendy or "hot".

Finally, parading his patients in cosmetic surgery fashion shows is the ultimate of hype and poor taste. A professional approach would be to introduce a prospective patient to one of his patients who has already undergone similar procedures

� **Please note: Websites A and B** have been created to exemplify strong and weak Internet presence, but neither one is a replica of an actual surgeon's website.

➤ Look for specifics about a surgeon's training, skill, credentials, artistic vision, scholarly contributions and concern for his patients. In the final analysis, you want someone with skilled hands and a heart that is in his work.

☞ Your first resource should be the Internet.

☞ Your second resource should be a phone call to the surgeon's nurse or office manager.

➤ Narrow your search and rule out the surgeons who don't meet important criteria <u>before</u> you schedule a single consultation.

☞ Try to get answers to all of the questions that appear on the *Sex, Lies and Cosmetic Surgery* CD-Part E, also reproduced on Pages 275-278 , <u>before</u> you schedule a consultation. That way, if you don't like the answers you receive, you need go no further and won't end up spending any of your hard earned money on an unnecessary consultation.

Appendix 5: Relaxation Techniques
Ways to Calm Your Mind

A number of highly respected researchers have published studies over the last several decades with compelling medical evidence in support of the physical benefits of calming one's mind. Collectively known as the *relaxation response*, these techniques cause blood pressure readings to drop, breathing rates to slow and muscles to become less tense.

Remember, a relaxed state of mind can significantly impact not just your healing, but your surgical results as well. If you are feeling stressed, here are four relaxation techniques which can do wonders to calm those jittery nerves.

> ➤ **Paced respiration** is one effective technique that takes little practice. Begin by inhaling slowly and deeply enough so that your abdomen is fully expanded. Say the number "five" silently to yourself as you exhale. Pause briefly, inhale slowly and deeply a second time and think "four" as you exhale. Continue at your own pace, counting down to "one". Repeat this cycle for 10 – 15 minutes.

> ➤ **Meditation** is an ancient practice used for centuries to evoke that relaxation response. Begin by selecting a word or simple phrase that is pleasing to you. (Some people choose a calming word or phrase from nature, religion or their belief system such as "trickling water" or "peace be with you".) Sit quietly

in a comfortable position and close your eyes. Relax your muscles, concentrating in turn on your feet, calves, thighs, abdomen, arms, fingers, chest, shoulders, neck and head. Breathe slowly and naturally, saying your chosen word or phrase to yourself each time you exhale. If other thoughts intrude, let them pass through without concern and return to your "mantra". Do this for a minimum of five minutes but ideally for ten to twenty minutes. For further assistance with meditation, see: **http://www.learningmeditation.com/room.htm**

➤ **Progressive muscle relaxation** is a technique first described by Edmund Jacobson, based on the premise that mental relaxation should naturally follow from physical relaxation. Lie on your back in a comfortable position in a quiet place free from all distractions. Tighten a muscle group in your feet, hold for five to eight seconds and then release and stay relaxed for fifteen to thirty seconds. Repeat this exercise as you gradually continue upward on your body to your legs, hips, pelvis, lower back, abdomen, neck, head, arms and hands. Each time, while releasing the tension, try to focus on the changes you feel when that muscle group is relaxed. Try to imagine stressful feelings flowing out of your body as you release each muscle group. With practice and time, progressive muscle relaxation helps you accurately identify tension signals in your own body and actively work to reduce stress and tension and their accompanying physical reactions. For more information on this technique, see: http://ourworld.compuserve.com/homepages/har/les1. htm

> **The Sanity Stone:** Dr. Millie Grenough, clinical instructor of psychiatry at the Yale University School of Medicine and author of *Oasis in the Overwhelm*, frequently introduces this simple stress reducing strategy during her executive training sessions. Hold a seashell, stone or other small object and focus all your attention on it. Notice its color, texture, pattern and other characteristics as you take 10 slow, deep breaths. Then gradually let your eyes and attention move out to your surroundings. Some of Millie's clients carry their serenity stones in their pockets and use them in typically stress producing situations such as traffic jams, before important business meetings, prior to initiating difficult conversations, etc.

Repetitive activities such as walking, playing a musical instrument, biking, knitting and Yoga are other ways to put yourself in a healthful state of mind.

Visit any of the following websites to read more about these and other techniques for stress reduction:

http://www.healthy.net/asp/templates/article.asp?PageType=article&ID=1205

http://health.discovery.com/ Once you arrive at this site, add: encyclopedias/3150.html
to the URL address box and press enter.

http://www.graduateresearch.com/reilly.htm

CR

Appendix 6: Internet and Book Resources
Where to Get Accurate Information About
Your Surgical Procedures:

➤ Most people feel more at ease once they have familiarized themselves with some basic information about their forthcoming surgical procedure(s).

➤ Knowledge gives you the tools to ask intelligent questions and communicate well with your surgeon and his staff.

❦ Internet Resources ❧

• **American Society for Aesthetic Plastic Surgery (ASAPS)**
URL: http://www.surgery.org/
This website will help you locate board certified plastic surgeons who are members of this prestigious society and it offers profiles about many of their members with links to their personal websites. You can click on *Procedures* to learn more about specific cosmetic surgical procedures or go to their *Photo Gallery* to view before and after photographs of individuals who have undergone cosmetic surgeries to various parts of the body. By entering their *Press Center*, you can read newsworthy articles relating to the field of cosmetic surgery, view current statistics, read descriptions of various procedures and more. Frequently asked questions and answers are listed, and you can also submit questions for consideration by ASAPS members.

• **American Society of Plastic Surgeons (ASPS)**
URL: http://www.plasticsurgery.org/
This website provides information on both reconstructive and cosmetic surgical procedures, informative articles on what's new in plastic surgery and patient stories about their plastic surgery experiences, categorized by specific procedure. The ASPS will help you locate an American board certified plastic surgeon in your area.

- **American Academy of Dermatological Surgery (AADS)**
URL: http://www.aboutskinsurgery.org/
This website will help you find a board certified dermatologic surgeon in the state or country of your choice. The patient section of this site provides a listing and brief description of the procedures performed by dermatologic surgeons, fact sheets about each procedure and before/after photographs.

- **The American Academy of Otolaryngology-Head and Neck Surgery (AAO)**
URL: http://www.entnet.org/
At present this website primarily is focused on non-cosmetic forms of head and neck surgeries.

- **The American Society of Ophthalmic Plastic and Reconstructive Surgery (ASOPRS)**
URL: http://www.asoprs.org/
This website provides information to define cosmetic and non-cosmetic eye conditions and the surgical procedures undertaken to correct them.

⋙ Cosmetic Surgery Support Groups ⋘

- **Implant Info by Nicole**
For more information about breast augmentation, go to http://www.ImplantInfo.com/, the world's largest and most popular Internet site for research about breast augmentation and breast implants. You will have access to other women's stories, personal experiences, an active chat room (visited by over ten thousand visitors daily), and before/after photographs of over 2000 women who have had breast augmentation surgery.

- **Facial Plastic Surgery Network**

For very thorough information about cosmetic surgical and non-surgical procedures of the face, eyes and neck, go to http://www.facialplasticsurgery.net. This site is both well organized and contains highly informative articles about each procedure. Their discussion area provides a forum for interacting with others considering surgery or in any post surgery stage of healing following any facial procedures. See before and after photographs at their photo gallery.

- **Liposite**

For more information about liposuction, go to: http://www.liposite.com, the sister site of Implant Info.com/, where you will find answers to those most frequently posed questions about liposuction. You can read about the personal experiences of others, view before and after photographs and join their online chat board.

❧ Other Cosmetic Surgery Resources ☙

- **Denise Thomas (Manhattan Cosmetic Surgery Consultant)**

Phone: 1-212-734-0233

URL: http://www.DeniseThomas.com/

If you do not have the time or inclination to do your own research, call Denise Thomas for recommendations for the best Manhattan based cosmetic surgeons.

- **Home Recovery:**

For shop-at-home convenience, check out their online catalogue at: http://www.homerecovery.com/ They have a wide assortment of post-surgical items that are well priced and thoughtfully designed. You will find just about anything you might want for your comfort or convenience while healing after surgery.

(e.g. a floppy hat with an attached scarf, a pillow with proper head elevation, special undergarments to wear after body surgery and more.).

❦ *Book Resources* ❧

There are many good books on cosmetic surgery, written from various medical perspectives. I have highlighted three below, each from the perspective of a different specialist: skin surgeries (Dermatologist), head and neck surgeries (ENT or Head and Neck Surgeon), full compliment of facial and body surgeries (Plastic Surgeon).

♦ **From a Board Certified Cosmetic Dermatologist**

Sundaram, Hema, M.D., *Face Value*, Living Planet Books, 2003.
Sundaram is a board certified cosmetic dermatologist who specializes in facial rejuvenation procedures. She explains procedures such as chemical peels, laser resurfacing, micro and macro dermabrasions, skin polishers and more. She also offers women who aren't entirely comfortable with "buying beauty" a calm and reasoned argument for the right to be beautiful. But Sundaram's book is something more than a rationale for cosmetic surgery. She discusses inner beauty as the secret to real outer beauty and offers guided meditations and principles of living: *Do at least one thing a day that inspires you*, tips on healthy living and other lifestyle changes that can slow your rate of aging. For those who choose to undergo cosmetic procedures, she shares some practical steps and encouragement for doing so. To highlight her expertise as a dermatologist, she presents a Seven-Minute at-home skin rejuvenation program. It was confirming for me to discover that Dr. Sundaram recommends the same Topix products to her patients that Michelle has made part of my daily routine.

♦ From a Board Certified Head and Neck Surgeon

Kotler, Robert, Md. *Secrets of A Beverly Hills Cosmetic Surgeon: The Experts Guide to Safe Successful Surgery,* **Ernest Mitchell Publishers, 2003.**

Dr. Kotler is a board certified Head and Neck Surgeon who specializes in cosmetic surgery restricted to those areas of the body. This book has been described as *the bible for the consumer who is looking for rejuvenation and is concerned about what procedure they really need* . . . Dr. Kotler's book is well formatted and easy to read and understand. Chapter 6 contains a photo gallery with an individual illustration and thumbnail description of each cosmetic facial and body procedure, some contributed by Dr. Kotler and others, by board certified plastic surgeons. Dr. Kotler makes a strong case for selecting the most experienced and narrowly focused specialist for the type surgery you are seeking.

♦ From a Board Certified Plastic Surgeon

Loftus, Jean M., M.D., *The Smart Woman's Guide to Plastic Surgery: Essential Information from a Female Plastic Surgeon,* **Contemporary Books, 2000.**

With clarity, precision and depth, this board certified plastic surgeon explains exactly what cosmetic plastic surgery can and cannot accomplish. Written in an inviting and understandable style, her book confronts issues such as: the hidden costs of cosmetic surgery and how to uncover them; telltale signs of cosmetic surgery and how to avoid them; medications that can ruin your results or lengthen your recovery; the difference between lasers, chemical peels, and dermabrasion - and how to determine which one is most appropriate for you; different techniques for facelifts and eyelid surgery, and why some work better than others; specifics about Botox, ultrasonic liposuction, tummy tucks, breast implants, thigh lifts, spider veins, age spots, permanent makeup; and just about everything else available in the cosmetic plastic surgery arena. From an overview of the different procedures to expectations, possible complications and recovery; this book offers an honest, ethical presentation of the field of cosmetic surgery.

Appendix 7: Associations, Boards and More

- **American Society for Aesthetic Plastic Surgery (ASAPS)**
Call 1-888-272-7711 to determine the membership status of any plastic surgeon. (See further information about the ASAPS in Appendix 6 under Internet Resources.)
URL: http://www.surgery.org/
Provides immediate references to ASAPS members who practice in the specific USA geographic area of your choice. This website posts informative articles, current statistics, descriptions of various procedures and more relating to the field of cosmetic surgery.

- **American Board of Medical Specialties (ABMS)**
URL: http://www.abms.org/
For topics of interest to both physicians and the public, this site will also tell you which medical specialties are actually recognized by the ABMS. For further information about the twenty-four medical specialties recognized by the ABMS, visit their website or call 1- 847-491-9091.

- **American Board of Plastic Surgery (ABPS)**
URL: http://www.abplsurg.org/
Call 1-215 587- 9322 to learn if a given surgeon is a board certified plastic surgeon. Their web site also provides background information on requirements for accreditation.

- **American Board of Otolaryngology (ABO)**
3050 Post Oak Road, Suite #1700, Houston, Texas 77056
Call 1-713-850-0399 to determine if your doctor is a board certified Otolaryngologist (ENT or Head and Neck Specialist).

- **American Board of Dermatology (ABD)**
URL: http//www.abderm.org
Email: abderm@hfhs.org
1-313- 874-1088

- **American Association for Accreditation of Ambulatory Surgery Facilities, Inc. (AAAASF)**
Call 1-888-545-5222 to determine if they have accredited the surgical facility used by your plastic surgeon.
URL: http://www.aaaaasf.org/
If your surgeon's facility has not been accredited by the AAAASF, call the next two accreditation associations on my list below (in the order provided):

- **Accreditation Association for Ambulatory Health Care (AAAHC)**
Call 1- 847-853-6060 to determine if they have accredited the surgical facility used by your plastic surgeon.
URL: http://www.aaahc.org/eweb/StartPage.aspx/

- **The Joint Commission on Accreditation of Healthcare Organizations (JCAHO)**, the major accrediting agency for hospitals.
Call 1- 630-792-5000 to determine if they have accredited the surgical facility used by your plastic surgeon.
URL: http://www.jcaho.org/

Appendix 8: Personal Profiles
More about the people whose names
appear in this book

☙ *Personal Profiles* ❧

Most of the interviews I conducted and all of the
questionnaire responses were from women who had
undergone some form of cosmetic surgery. For each of
these women, I accurately list her surgical procedures, age
and marital status at the time of her surgery; but it is likely
that I altered some of the other details to honor
confidentiality and protect her right to privacy. In all cases, I
have tried to maintain the essence of each individual while
writing her profile.

I have also included in this appendix the names of
professionals in allied fields working with cosmetic surgery
patients: (anesthesiologists, estheticians, psychologists, a
Nurse Practitioner/First Assist and Registered Nurses), all of
whom I consulted to help clarify, expand or otherwise help
me gain needed perspectives.

All names that follow, listed in alphabetical order, became
an integral part of this book through their valued input.

**Now please meet the wonderful people for have
contributed to *Sex, Lies and Cosmetic Surgery*.**

Abby is a thirty-three year old woman whom I met at a conference. When she told me she had *little tolerance for those who indulge in such activities,* I laughed as I said that she might feel differently in about twenty years. When I asked her if she would like to include a statement of her thoughts in my book, she readily agreed.
(A story contributed by ABBY appears in Chapter 12.)

Alan M. Kisner, MD. a Fellow of the American College of Surgeons, board certified by The American Board of Plastic Surgery, maintains an active private practice in New York City and Huntington, Long Island. (More about Dr. Kisner's professional contributions and background can be found on the bottom of page 225-226.)
Born and raised in Johannesburg, South Africa, Dr. Kisner has maintained close ties to his family's homeland. Son of a distinguished urologist and world class artist, Dr. Kisner inherited many of his father's special talents as he pursued his unique interest in the aesthetics of plastic surgery. He earned his undergraduate degree at Witwatersrand University, an institution that has made its mark nationally and internationally, with an alumni list that includes Nelson Mandela and four Nobel laureates. He and his wife, Dawn Kisner, own the exclusive Makweti Safari Lodge in the Limpopo Province of South Africa. He has been an active participant in a South African project to return a hunting area to the wild.

Alfina is a former high school English teacher of outstanding intellect. The other members of my *Reading Hours* book group have been ever appreciative of her contribution as one of our members. She is admired not just for her perceptive observations, but for the respect and interest she shows for other points of view.
(A story contributed by ALFINA appears in Chapter 9.)

Alice is a beauty consultant and cosmetologist who speaks of *looking good* as essential in her line of work, so she views cosmetic surgery as more necessity than indulgence. She lives in a rural area of Conn. raising pedigreed poodles for ultimate adoption, both to supplement her income and to satisfy her love of animals.

Procedures: Breast lift: Age 47; Eyes, lower face lift; Age 50; Marital status: Married
(A story contributed by ALICE appears in Chapter 9.)

Alex is Jean Posillico's son. (See below.) I interviewed Alex to listen first hand to a son's reaction to his mother's cosmetic surgery.

(A story contributed by ALEX appears in Chapter 9.)

Alisa
Procedures: Breast lift, thigh lift, tummy tuck; Age: 47; Marital status: Divorced
(The stories about ALISA that appear in Chapters 7 and 9 were contributed by Denise Thomas.)

Amy: A profile about Amy is embedded into the text of Chapter 6: *You Might Fall in Love With Your Plastic Surgeon.*
Procedures: Facelift, brow lift, neck, eyes; Age: 57; Marital status: Married
(A story contributed by AMY appears in Chapter 6.)

Anesthesiologist: A prominent Manhattan cosmetic surgery anesthesiologist contributed her expertise to Chapter 10, *Misperceptions and Misconceptions,* but asked to remain anonymous.

Anne (pronounced Ann) is a refined, soft-spoken woman from Harrisburg, Pennsylvania. Slim and petite, with highlighted chestnut brown hair worn at chin length, she has that fair skinned complexion and hazel green eyes that define Irish beauties. Anne is a Registered Nurse employed at a major hospital near her home. She and her husband enjoy many activities together including joint workouts at a local gym. Anne tells me she is a voracious reader and someday hopes to write some women's fiction. Her hobbies include knitting, needle arts, gardening and home decorating.

Procedures: Facelift, neck, eyes; Age: 55; Marital status: Married
(Stories contributed by ANNE appear in Chapters 1, 3, 7, 9, 10 and Appendix 9: Additional stories for Chapters 7 and 10.)

335

Anne (pronounced Annie) Burke has had vast experience within the field of plastic surgery. Having worked with three plastic surgeons during the past fourteen years, she has gained knowledge with each position, from patient coordinator to patient-physician liaison. Aside from her family and career, her greatest loves are her golden retriever, Watson, and her three cats.
(Stories about **Annie** appear in my Epilogue.)

Arlene is a friend and former colleague, who sent me a savvy comment that appears in Chapter 9, *Secrecy, Deception and Lies.*

Augusta, a more recent addition to my neighborhood, brings lots of energy and humor to my life. This Brazilian beauty is the mother of two talented girls who come first in her list of priorities, with tennis and Yoga two of her additional passions.
(A story about AUGUSTA appears in Chapter 9.)

Barbara is in her mid twenties and describes her current boyfriend as her *first really committed relationship.* She is a serious minded young woman who teaches English literature at a competitive high school in Manhattan. She holds a Master's Degree in her area of interest and hopes to pursue a PhD. to enable her to eventually teach on a college level.
Procedures: Liposuction of legs and thighs; Age: 23; Marital status: Single
(Stories contributed by BARBARA appear in Chapter 9 and Appendix 9: Additional stories for Chapter 7.)

Beauty is a Manhattan based cosmetic surgery nurse/esthetician, whom I promised complete anonymity because of the extreme sensitivity of the information she supplied.
(Stories contributed by BEAUTY appear in Chapter 6.)

'Beauty Queen' is a Questionnaire Respondent. She listed psychic development, healing through Reiki and writing a book as her special interests and her children, her most important achievement. She had eye surgery to eliminate puffiness and bags, but felt that this one procedure made considerable improvement to her overall appearance. She attributes her deeper involvement in her special interest pursuits at least in part to her post surgery *greatly increased self-esteem.* She checked off: *I tend to be more candid and revealing in my conversations,* another characteristic of increased self-esteem, as the statement that best describes her post surgery responses to others.
Procedures: eyes; Age: 49; Marital status: Married
(A story contributed by BEAUTY QUEEN appears in Chapter 6.)

Beth
(The story about Beth that appears in Chapter 1 was contributed by Katie.)

Betsy is a school administrator in a Boston suburb, mother of two sons and a recent first time grandmother. Her penchant for golf and ballroom dancing speak volumes about her energetic style – so much so that she claims the hardest part of her surgical recovery was staying put at home. After her surgical healing was complete, she placed an updated picture of herself on the Internet and has received *more responses than she can handle.* She is attracted to men who enjoy active pursuits as walking in the city or visiting museums and to those who are open to adventure. She describes couch potato types as "not for me". Betsy loves visiting Sedona, Arizona for its picturesque beauty, but hopes to one day soon take a trip to Australia, New Zealand and the Fiji Islands.
Procedures: Facelift, eyes, neck, fat injections; Age: 57; Marital status: Divorced
(A story contributed by BETSY appears in Chapter 6.)

Bobbi is a long time friend whom I designated a member of my control group. *(See Additional Stories to my Epilogue in Appendix 9 for an explanation of this fun experiment.)* Normally game to try something new, Bobbi is hardly a person I would describe as overly conventional, yet when I confided in her that I was going to have a facelift, I nearly had to lift her off the floor. This was one announcement she never would have predicted from me. Bobbi is a collector of craft pins and necklaces.
(A story about BOBBI appears in Appendix 9: Lois' Story 3 in Additional stories for Chapter 9.)

Carmella is a young woman who enjoys leisure time activities of ballroom dancing and painting. A Reading Specialist in a large mid-western school district, Carmella has earned a Professional Diploma in her area of expertise and has done extensive research on how the brain develops and works for all ages. She describes herself as *a good conversationalist who enjoys the company of others*. A motivational speaker, Carmella helps other individuals prepare for interviews and locate new jobs. She tells me that her eyes are her prettiest feature.
Procedures: Tummy tuck, liposuction; Age: 32; Marital status: Single (Stories contributed by CARMELLA appear in Chapters 8 and 9.)

Carol is a woman whose feet never seem to touch the ground. She doesn't just participate in activities, she dives into them head first, often landing in leadership roles. When she joined her Retired Teachers Association, she soon became their president. When she joined an investment club, she soon led that group as their senior partner. A retired math teacher from a prominent Nassau County, Long Island school district, Carol is hardly retired from life. When not babysitting for one of her eight grandchildren, she is more likely to be spotted on a golf course, competing in a tennis tournament, skiing down a Colorado ski slope or off on a Elderhostel trip with one of her friends or grandchildren. Closer to home, she teaches Sunday School and plays the bells for her local church, takes tap dance and bridge lessons, volunteers at a residence for troubled young women and more. I wonder if she ever sleeps!

Procedures: Facelift, eyes, microdermabrasion; Age: 63; Marital status: Widowed
(Stories contributed by CAROL appear in Chapters 3, 7, 8 and 9.)

Carole is my daughter-in-law Kristen's mother. Although she never had cosmetic surgery herself, she offered words of encouragement and sound advice as she guided me in my search for a plastic surgeon.

(CAROLE's story appears in my Epilogue.)

Chesty is a respondent to my Cosmetic Surgery Questionnaire. A music teacher by profession, this young woman experienced *life altering* positive impacts to her surgery with dramatic boosts to her self-esteem, sexual functioning and overall level of happiness.

Procedures: Breast augmentation; Age: 29; Marital status: Single
(Stories contributed by CHESTY appear in Chapters 1, 3 and 7.)

Cindy
(A story about Cindy that appears in Chapter 1 was contributed by Denise Thomas.)
Procedures: Facelift, eyes, neck, brow lift; Age: 52; Marital status: Married

Cookie Levy is a cosmetic surgery Registered Nurse, with seventeen years of experience in both the Operating Room and in aftercare with cosmetic surgery patients. I consulted with Cookie on some of the finer points of surgery and recovery. She carefully reviewed my timeline checklists and amended them with eight suggestions of her own.

(Stories contributed by COOKIE appear in my Epilogue and in the Timeline Checklist, which appears as Part H on the *Sex, Lies and Cosmetic Surgery* CD.)

Dani
Procedures: Facelift, eyes, browlift; Age: 61; Marital status: Widowed and Remarried
(The story about Dani that appears in Chapter 1 was contributed by Dorothy Birnham.)

David B. Sarwer, Ph.D, Associate Professor of Psychology in the Departments of Psychiatry and Surgery at the University of Pennsylvania School of Medicine, is a consultant to the Edwin and Fannie Gray Hall Center for Human Appearance. Internationally known for his research on the psychological aspects of cosmetic and reconstructive plastic surgery, he regularly presents his research at meetings of the American Society of Plastic Surgeons and has testified before the Food and Drug Administration on the psychological aspects of breast implants. Dr. Sarwer is the lead editor of *Psychological Aspects of Reconstructive and Cosmetic Plastic Surgery: Clinical, Empirical, and Ethical Perspectives* (Lippincott, Williams, and Wilkens, 2006), the only text of its kind to summarize the research on the psychological aspects of plastic surgery. In addition to his research, he maintains an active clinical practice in which he treats individuals with a range of appearance concerns. Dr. Sarwer was awarded his Bachelor's Degree Summa Cum Laude, Phi Beta Kappa from Tulane University in 1990. He received his Master's Degree in 1992 and doctorate in clinical psychology in 1995, both from Loyola University Chicago.

Dawn accepted her mother's offer of a gift of cosmetic surgery despite her husband's protestations. Her surgery was a success, but precipitated the unraveling of an already fragile marriage.
Procedures: Tummy tuck, Liposuction; Age: Childbearing age; Marital status: Divorced
(A story contributed by DAWN appears in Chapter 9.)

Dee is a veterinary assistant who tells me that since as long as she can remember she has had a passion for all four legged creatures. By age seven she had decided to stop eating meat and before adolescence had become a strict vegetarian. She opted for early marriage instead of pursuing a post graduate degree, but has learned so much *just working in the field and assuming gradual responsibilities beyond*

what most any assistants would do, that she is quite certain she could pass the exams without matriculating, if allowed to do so. **Dee** lives in Brooklyn Heights, but commutes to Manhattan daily via an express bus.
Procedures: Facelift, liposuction; Age: 56; Marital status: Divorced
(A story contributed by DEE appears in Chapter 9.)

Denise Thomas, Manhattan Cosmetic Surgery Consultant, contributed as an *at large* consultant to many chapters of this book. A complete profile of Denise, including her beautiful picture, can be found in Appendix 1, page 301 of this book.

Diane, a slim woman with highlights in her dark blond hair, stands 5' 7". She describes herself as *generous in her friendships*. When I asked her to explain that statement further, she told me that friends are very important to her. Widowed at age forty-eight, she has remained close to her mother-in-law and other members of her husband's family, in addition to *an excellent support group of friends and relatives*. Each summer she goes on a one week *girls' vacation* with her daughter, mother, sister and niece. Diane loves to read, play tennis, compete in her bowling league and spend extended weekends at her summer beach home. She volunteers twice a week with Hospice Care.
Procedures: Nose: age 16, Facelift and eyes: age 56; Marital status: Widowed
(Stories contributed by DIANE appear in Chapters 3, 7, 9 and Appendix 9: Additional stories for Chapter 10.)

Donna is a dental assistant who has used her long time fascination for puppets to wonderful advantage as she assists the pediatric dentist with whom she works. She usually meets each new child/patient first, talking through the voice of one of her puppets, to relax and help the child feel at ease. She is apparently quite an asset because the dentist keeps *making me new offers I can't refuse whenever I speak about retirement.*
Procedures: Facelift, eyes; Age: 59; Marital status: Married
(Stories contributed by DONNA appear in Chapter 7 and Appendix 9: Additional stories for Chapter 7.)

Dorothy Birnham, the former Director of Voluntary Action on Long Island, now lives in a popular retirement community near the tri city area of North Carolina. She contributed to this book through several in-depth interviews, which included both her personal reasons for not undergoing cosmetic surgery and stories about several of her women friends who did make that decision for themselves.
(Stories contributed by DOROTHY appear in Chapters 1, 3 and 8.)

Edith is Gladwyn's mother. (See below.) We met by chance at the theatre and discovered a common thread in our lives. Our conversation elicited one pertinent story that appears in the Epilogue of this book.

Elizabeth lives in NYC and is the mother of a teenage daughter, whom she and her late husband adopted after many childless years. Several years after her husband's death, she met a pilot and is *loving life once again.*
Procedures: Facelift, eyes, neck; Age: 51; Marital status: Widowed
(The stories about ELIZABETH that appear in Chapters 4 and 7 were contributed by Denise Thomas.)

Evelyn is a personal friend who unwittingly became a member of my 'experimental group'. *(See Appendix 9 for an explanation of this fun experiment.)* Evelyn is a realtor who has so much energy and enthusiasm for her work that it is little wonder she is a top 1% producer for her company. She and I became grandmothers within weeks of one another. Soon thereafter we began to arrange toddler play dates, which gave us both more opportunities to beam with delight.
(A story about EVELYN appears in Appendix 9: Additional stories for my Epilogue.)

Fran Orgovan is a clinical esthetician and NY State licensed teacher of esthetics who has worked with several renown plastic surgeons. She has added her expertise to this book both as a consultant and as a cosmetic surgery patient. **Fran** is Justin Orgovan's mother. (See below.)
Procedures: Tummy tuck, Breast lift, eyes

(Stories contributed by FRAN appear in Chapters 3, 4, 9, 10, and 12.)

Gail, a professional singer, has a voice so versatile that she is equally at home with disco and light opera. She has performed on stages across the United States and occasionally, in European cities including London and Paris. She describes herself as a tall, willowy brunette, happily married to a musician who shares her love for all things musical. When not traveling or performing, Gail says she prefers to stay home and dabble in the kitchen, preparing a special meal to enjoy solo with her husband or with a close, small circle of friends. Gail's charming, somewhat reticent personality seemed a bit of a contradiction to some of her interview contributions. They always say to watch out for the quiet ones!
Procedures: Facelift, brow lift, neck, eyes; Age: 58; Marital status: Married
(Stories contributed by GAIL appear in Chapters 1, 3, 6, 12 and Appendix 9: Additional stories for Chapter 6.)

Gina, a retired middle school teacher with special talents in math and science, is now affiliated with a university group involved with programs for lifelong learning, where she concentrates on courses focused on art history, music and poetry writing. She has four grandchildren whom she visits frequently and speaks of them as *additional blessings in her rich, full life.* She and her husband recently purchased a small apartment in southern Florida, to join the other Snowbirds in escaping the brutal northern winters of New Hampshire.
Procedures: Facelift, eyes, neck; Age: 62; Marital status: Married
(Stories contributed by GINA appear in Chapters 1, 3, 4 and Appendix 9: Additional stories for Chapter 1.)

Gladwyn is a Professor of Pathology at Fletcher Allen Health Care in Burlington, Vermont. We met by chance at the theatre and discovered a common thread in our lives. She is Edith's daughter. (See above.) A story about Gladwyn appears in the Epilogue of this book.

Grace is a sales representative for a cosmeceutical company whose products are available through the trade only. Her clients include dermatologists, plastic surgeons and estheticians. **Grace** hails from Staten Island, NY, and enjoys its outdoor environment. She occupies her leisure time with running, walking, cross country skiing and playing ball with her retriever at the local dog park. She has one married daughter living out of state and a son currently completing his last year of law school.

Procedures: Facelift, eyes; Age: 50; Marital status: Divorced
(Stories contributed by GRACE appear in Chapters 9 and 12.)

Harriet Spitzer is one of the women I interviewed who did not want to consider cosmetic surgery for herself, and brings that other perspective to light in this book. A profile about Harriet is embedded into the text of Chapter 8: *What Deters Us?*

(Stories contributed by HARRIET S. appear in Chapters 8, 9 and 12)

Harriet W. has never had cosmetic surgery, but was a great support for me when I had mine. I designated her a member of my 'control' group. *(See Appendix 9: Additional Stories to my Epilogue for an explanation of this fun experiment.)* I couldn't have asked for better support people than she and her husband, Joel, who were there for me with encouragement and enthusiasm from start to finish. They enjoy many activities together including travel and genealogy.

(Stories contributed by Harriet W. appear in Chapter 9 and the Epilogue.)

Hartley is a respondent to my Cosmetic Surgery Questionnaire. Although post surgery healing took longer than she had anticipated, on a scale of 1-5 (with 1 being the lowest and 5 the highest), she rated her satisfaction as 5, and said it has made her *feel younger, more energetic and happier*. She recognizes that she now radiates those feelings in her interactions with others. Hartley lives in a suburban

community, is the mother of three grown children and grandmother to four. She describes herself as a *family oriented, outgoing and extroverted - a person who enjoys golf, Pilates, bridge, stitching and eating out with friends.*
Procedures: Facelift: Age: 56; Eyes: Age: 58; Marital status: Married
(A story contributed by HARTLEY appears in Chapter 6.)

Hewitt had read about my study in the Barnard Alumnae Magazine, tried to complete my questionnaire, which was then posted on a private Internet site, but ran into a computer glitch. She called me to talk about her difficulty, but then never went on to complete the questionnaire. Consequently I know little about her other than that she once hailed from Manhattan, now lives in Florida and is a long term survivor of ovarian cancer.
Procedures: Neck and liposuction under the chin; Age: 60+; Marital status: Married
(Stories contributed by HEWITT appear in Chapter 7 and Appendix 9: Additional stories for Chapter 10.)

Hope, a respondent to my Cosmetic Surgery Questionnaire, said she experienced a minimum of discomfort during recovery following surgery and healed at the rate she had anticipated. On a scale of 1-5 (with 1 being the lowest and 5 the highest), she rated her overall satisfaction with her surgical results as 5 and claims that it has made her feel *happier, more content and somewhat more sensual*. As an aside, she noted that men have shown a *more overt interest* since her surgery. Hope lists *confidence in her abilities, love from another person* and *feeling productive* as the ingredients that give her a positive self-image, with physical appearance further down on the list. Hope has initiated body building exercises since her surgery and expressed special interests in reading, music and golf. She further described herself as *a good teacher* and *nurturer of her family*.
Procedures: Facelift, eyes; Age: 61; Marital status: Married
(Stories contributed by HOPE appear in Chapter 6, 10 and Appendix 9: Additional stories for Chapter 3.)

Jane, a woman living in the suburbs of Chicago, takes pride in both her professional accomplishments and her physical appearance. Although thoroughly dedicated to her work as a high school administrator, she is also tuned to personal care and grooming. Jane dresses fashionably, uses the bimonthly services of an esthetician and exercises at a local gym at least three times per week. Married for over thirty years, she and her husband recently celebrated the wedding of their eldest child. Together they enjoy the leisure time activities of golf, weather permitting, theatre and concerts.
Procedures: Facelift, eyes, fat injections; Age: 57; Marital status: Married
(Stories contributed by JANE appear in Chapters 7, 9 and 10 and Appendix 9: Additional stories for Chapters 9 and 10.)

Janet
(The story about JANET that appears in Chapter 7 was contributed by Denise Thomas.)
Procedures: Facelift, neck; Age: 47; Marital status: Divorced

Janine is an airline flight attendant, who says she loves the adventure of travel and still has at least thirty-two dots on her map of places she wants to visit.
Procedures: Breast lift, Tummy tuck; Age: 37; Marital status: Married
(A story contributed by JANINE appears in Chapter 7.)

Jean Posillico, registered nurse/clinical esthetician and mother of Alex Posillico, (See above.). **Jean** contributed both as a consultant and cosmetic surgery patient.
Procedures: Breast reduction; Age:39; Marital status: Married
(Stories contributed by JEAN appear in Chapter 9 and Chapter 10.

Jennifer, an announcer for an Arizona radio station, generally covers the daily headlines and weather forecasts. She has a particular interest in politics, which she interweaves into her aired segments *at every appropriate moment*
Procedures: Facelift, eyes; Age: 48; Marital status: Single

Jenny Jasper is one of the women I interviewed who did not choose cosmetic surgery for herself, who brings that other perspective to this book. A profile about Jenny is embedded into the text of Chapter 8: *What Deters Us?* An early reader of my manuscript, Jenny offered several thought provoking suggestions.
(Stories contributed by JENNY appear in Chapter 8.)

Joan has never had any cosmetic surgery, but had some interesting reactions to mine. A gourmet cook, avid bicyclist and devoted gardener, she devours the New York Times daily and remembers all the details of its editorials. You have to be on your toes when you converse with Joan or play opposite her on the tennis court, where she packs away a strong crosscourt shot.
(A story about JOAN contributed by this author appears in Appendix 9: Additional stories for Chapter 9.)

'Jockette' is a respondent to my Cosmetic Surgery Questionnaire, who experienced considerable pain after the microdermabrasion procedure around her mouth and found that healing time was prolonged. She has learned her lesson and now wears sunscreen on a daily basis. 'Jockette' reported on the many post surgery compliments she has received about her appearance, but that she has not experienced any emotional impacts such as increased self-esteem or changes to her overall level of happiness. She notes *love from another person* and *confidence in my abilities* as key contributors to her feelings of positive self-image.
Procedures: Facelift, eyes, microdermabrasion; Age: 63; Marital status: Widowed
(Stories contributed by JOCKETE appear in Chapter 6 and Appendix 2.)

Jolie
· **(The stories about JOLIE that appear in Chapter 1 and in Appendix 9: Additional stories for Chapter 1 were contributed by Denise Thomas.)**

Jody
(The stories about JODY that appear in Appendix 9: Additional stories for Chapters 1 and 4 were contributed by Denise Thomas.)

Joyce
(The story about JOYCE that appears in Chapter 4 was contributed by Denise Thomas.)
Procedures: Facelift, eyes, neck, nose; Age: 53; Marital status: Divorced

Judith is a retired Special Education teacher who lives in Manhattan. We connected through a mutual friend and spoke by telephone. She described herself as *tall and thin, a person who always had a good self-image, dresses well and maintains flattering hairstyles.* Last year Judith was seriously ill and needed kidney surgery. After being faced with a serious illness, she describes a facelift as *kind of frivolous* by comparison.
Procedures: Facelift, lower eyes, jowls, neck; Age: 63; Marital status: Divorced
(Stories contributed by JUDITH appear in Chapter 9 and Appendix 9: Additional stories for Chapters 7 and 9.)

Judy, effervescent and full of fun, is ready to have a good time at a moment's notice. When you meet her, what you see first are her sparkling eyes and a warm smile. She and I first got to know one another on the beaches of Cancun, Mexico where she and her girlfriend, both single women at the time, took daily, bikini clad strolls near the shore line, hoping to meet up with something more than sea shells! When they left Cancun, they headed straight for the ski slopes of Colorado. She and her college roommate once drove cross country in bathing suits, occasionally pool hopping while traveling through those hot climates states. Judy still loves the beach, but now shares it more sedately - with her husband - in their winter condo on the West Coast of Florida. Her gregarious nature enabled her to wrangle an invitation to a private party held for Elvis Presley some years ago. Judy's career as an interior designer seems well suited to her personality. But there is also a serious side to this wonderful woman, as you surely have determined after reading the story of her bout with breast cancer.

Procedures: Breast reconstruction; Age: 52; Marital status: Married
(Stories contributed by JUDY appear in Chapters 1, 3, 6 and Appendix 9: Additional stories for Chapter 6.)

Julie: A profile about Julie is embedded into the text of Chapter 6: *You Might Fall in Love With Your Plastic Surgeon.*
Procedures: Upper and lower eye lifts; Age: 42; Marital status: Widowed
(Stories contributed by JULIE appear in Chapter 6 and Appendix 9: Additional stories for Chapter 6.)

Justin is Fran Orgovan's son, (See above.), whom I interviewed to listen first hand to a son's reaction to his mother's cosmetic surgery.
(A story contributed by JUSTIN appears in Chapter 9.)

Katherine lives in a suburban New Jersey community and commutes to her work as an investment banker in Manhattan. She loves looking younger and notices that the men at work have suddenly become more attentive. Her only child is now completing her college education. Once this big expense is put to rest, Katherine hopes to travel to safe regions of the mid east.
Procedures: Facelift, brow lift, eyes; Age: 46; Marital status: Divorced
(A story contributed by KATHERINE appears in Chapter 9.)

Katie, a hairstylist with a devoted clientele, self-described as *a vivacious blond*, is a part time Yoga teacher, alternate weekend personal trainer. I felt enormous energy and confidence from her during our telephone conversation, where she also spoke about how comfortable she was amongst men. No wonder! She grew up as the only girl in a family with six brothers. **Katie** is not the type to be easily embarrassed or intimidated. Nonetheless, this Chicago woman with the bubbling personality, lowered her voice to a murmur as she read some of those Internet responses to her posted question about her post surgery increased feelings of sensuality.

Procedures: Breast lift, liposuction; Age: 43; Marital status: Single

(Stories contributed by KATIE appear in Chapters 1 and 4.)

Kelly lives in an urban environment, but otherwise asked to remain anonymous.

Procedures: Breast augmentation, eyes; Age: 52; Marital status: Married

(Stories contributed by KELLY appear in Chapter 3 and Appendix 9: Additional stories for Chapter 3.)

Kristen works as a corporate trainer for that ever-evolving field of computer technology. She is outsourced to various corporations to instruct their employees on software applications pertinent to their work. She and her husband live outside of Boston, Ma., where they are able to take advantage of the many cultural opportunities offered within their city. They own a small summer cottage in the Berkshires where they enjoy the surrounding culture of musical concerts and summer stock theatre.

Procedures: Facelift, eyes, neck; Age: 49; Marital status: Married

(A story contributed by KRISTEN appears in Chapter 7.)

Laura

(The story about LAURA that appears in Chapter 9 was contributed by Denise Thomas.)

Procedures: Facelift, eyes, neck; Age: 47; Marital status: Divorced

Lauren, an interior designer specializing in the redefinition and optimization of one's commercial workspace, counts many physicians and attorneys from her hometown of Atlanta, Georgia as her clients. This outgoing, hazel eyed blond enjoys volunteer work, both at her church, where she plays the organ for special occasions, and at a local hospital, where she entertains children by playing popular songs for them on her harmonica. **Lauren's** daughter shares her

favorite hobby of flower arranging. Her two sons share her love of mystery and science fiction books, which lead to many lively discussions amongst the three of them.
Procedures: Facelift, neck, eyes; Age: 50; Marital status: Divorced
(Stories contributed by LAUREN appear in Chapters 1, 7, 9, 10 and Appendix 9: Additional stories for Chapters 7 and 10.)

Lee and her husband abandoned suburbia for a beautiful country home in Vermont. Lee is an avid gardener, reader and all round warm, friendly person. She has never had cosmetic surgery, but had some interesting reactions to mine.
(A story about LEE appears in Appendix 9: Additional stories for Chapter 9.)

Leo R. McCafferty, M.D., a Fellow of the American College of Surgeons, is a board certified plastic surgeon certified by The American Board of Plastic Surgery, who maintains an active private practice in Pittsburgh, Pa. A member of the American Society for Aesthetic Plastic Surgery (ASAPS) and At-Large Member of their Board of Directors (2004-2007), he is also a member of the American Society of Plastic Surgeons (ASPS) and Clinical Assistant Professor of Plastic Surgery at the University of Pittsburgh School of Medicine. Dr. McCafferty has served as Plastic Surgeon for the men's and women's professional U.S. Open Golf Championships and is Plastic Surgery Consultant to the Pittsburgh Steelers. He received his Bachelor of Science degree from Penn State University, his Medical Doctorate from Temple University, his internship and residency in General Surgery at Cedars-Sinai Medical Center in Los Angeles, California and his training in Plastic Surgery at the University of Miami/Jackson Memorial Medical Center in Miami, Florida .

Lily
Procedures: Facelift, neck, eyes, nose; Age: 53; Marital status: Divorced
(The story about LILY that appears in Chapter 6 was contributed by Denise Thomas.)

Linda Gottlieb, originally an Operating Room nurse, went for advanced training to become a Nurse Practitioner and First Assistant. Eventually she decided to specialize in cosmetic plastic surgery nursing, a field that compliments her artistic bent. **Linda** has not personally undergone cosmetic surgery, but says that one thing she has learned about life is: *We should never say never about anything.*
(Stories about LINDA appear in the Epilogue of this book.)

Linda Novick is another of the women I interviewed who did not want to consider cosmetic surgery for herself, who brings that other perspective to light in this book. A profile about Linda is embedded into the text of Chapter 8: *What Deters Us?* Linda now winters in Florida, but manages to return to LI often enough to join most of our Reading Hours book group sessions.
(The story about LINDA that appears in Chapter 8 resulted from a lengthy interview and follow-up e-mail messages between the two of us.)

Liza
(The story about LIZA that appears in Chapter 1 was contributed by Katie.)

Lorraine Schles-Esposito, Ph.D., is a psychologist, former colleague and friend. Our professional relationship provided us with daily opportunities to interact in many stimulating and productive ways. I admired her deep commitment to the children of our school district, her perseverance and her enthusiasm for life, even during times of adversity. During these last several years, she has been reorienting herself from career pursuits to devotion to a newly blended family, which she describes as "an act of love". Active in tennis and golf, as well as the social community of Admiral's Cove, it is no

surprise to anyone that Lorraine now heads various committees and is captain of her tennis team.
(LORRAINE contributed her professional expertise to Chapters 5 and 8.)

Louise
(A story about LOUISE (from Louisiana) appears in Chapter 1.)

Lucy describes herself as *rather introverted* and says she spends part of each day *with* her nose in a book. A dedicated hospital volunteer, she has recently gravitated to the children's wing where she has found her special niche as "the lady with the magic box". This box contains special projects she has designed to engage the children, as Origami (Japanese paper folding) and magic tricks. She likes to leave the children with something related to the project-of-the-day so they can continue to master their skills after she is gone. She and her husband enjoy social dancing and travel.
Procedures: Facelift, eyes, laser resurfacing; Age: 54; Marital status: Married
(Stories contributed by LUCY appear in Chapters 4 and 7.)

Lucille
(A story contributed by LUCILLE appears in Chapter 10.)

'Makeover' is a Questionnaire Respondent who, on a scale of 1-5 (with 5 being the highest), rated her surgical results as 5. Although these results made her feel *happier and more self-confident*, she does not believe that surgery changed her overall feelings about herself. She is the mother of two children and grandmother to two as well. **'Makeover'** described herself as *family and relationship oriented, outgoing and extroverted with liberal values and thoughts.*
Procedures: Chin implant, nose; Age 54; Facelift, brows; Age: 63; Marital status: Married
(Stories contributed by 'MAKEOVER' appear in Chapters 6 and 10.)

Maria is an elementary school teacher who had her cosmetic surgery during summer vacation. She confides that she sometimes manages to get in an hour of her favorite leisure time activity, tennis, before her 8:30 AM sign-in at school. She works in a prominent school district on LI, NY and asked that no further details be listed to identify her.
Procedures: Tummy tuck; Age: 32; Marital status: Single
(Stories contributed by MARIA appear in Chapter 10 and Appendix 9: Additional stories for Chapter 10.)

Marie Gemma is a Registered Nurse, neighbor and friend. We have lived next door to one another for over thirty years and have maintained a close friendship for many reasons, including the fact that our shared mutual respect includes respect for privacy. Once a month we meet for breakfast and conversation, discussing nearly everything short of politics, the one topic on which we occasionally disagree! If I were limited to four words to describe **Marie**, I would name: *thoughtful, competent, devoted* and *caring*.
(MARIE contributed her professional expertise to Chapter 10 and to my Epilogue.)

Marilyn is a law professor who recently accepted a position at a southern university in order to relocate to a warmer climate. Her new colleagues never saw her before her facelift and surmise that she is in her forties. Marilyn is aware of their faulty assumptions because they continually advise her about the proper steps she should take to assure herself of being granted tenure, without any inkling that she plans to retire in less than the six years required to become a tenured professor.
Procedures: Facelift, eyes, neck, liposuction of neck; Age: 56; Marital status: Married
(Stories contributed by MARILYN appear in Chapters 9, 10 and Appendix 9: Additional stories for Chapters 9 and 10.)

MaryLou is a Cosmetic Surgery Questionnaire Respondent who reported that both of her cosmetic surgeries were *an enormous boost to her self-esteem and her ability to function as a sexual human being.* Her most telling comment was: "Why didn't I do this sooner?"
Procedures: Breast reduction: Age: 42; liposuction of thighs; Age: 43; Marital status: Divorced
(Stories contributed by MaryLou appear in Chapter 7 and Appendix 9: Additional stories for Chapter 7.)

Michelle Martel, also known as *The Duchess of Dermis,* is a brilliant esthetician who has gained her expertise while working under the guidance of several eminent dermatologists and plastic surgeons. She has the energy of six people and enthusiasm enough to share with them all. A woman of many talents, marvelous wit and a candid, uninhibited manner, she adds a refreshing spark to any ordinary day. But Michelle's fun loving nature hardly captures the essence of this woman who firmly believes in the beauty of the soul, but also has a deep respect for modern cosmetic technology and its power to bring harmony to the human spirit. Michelle was one of the first people to explore the potential of light and laser technology, and is respected as one of the leaders in dual modality laser techniques (different wave lengths), to treat a wide range of cosmetic needs, adjustments and enhancements. A holistic practitioner, Michelle treats both body and soul with equal dedication.
(Stories contributed by MICHELLE appear in Chapter 2 as well as my Introduction, Epilogue and Afterwords.)

Nancy lives in a rural setting of wide open spaces in upstate New York. A pet enthusiast, her family consists of a husband, three teenage children, two Golden Retrievers, four kittens, a momma cat, two caged guinea pigs and a parakeet – all of whom share their inside space. Outside, two horses reside in their backyard barn. Not surprisingly, horseback riding is Nancy's favorite leisure time activity. A skilled jumper, Nancy occasionally enters local competitions along with her children.

Procedures: Breast reduction; Age: 43; Marital status: Married

(Stories contributed by Nancy appear in Chapter 3 and Appendix 9: Additional stories for Chapter 7.)

Nicole is a young mother who lives in southern Florida with her husband and two small children. She described her body build as "slender but curvy". Her husband helped her do exhaustive research prior to her surgery and encouraged her to start an Internet support group for other women. ImplantInfo.com/ was the first such site and has grown into the most active Internet resource for women undergoing breast augmentation procedures. She has been an advocate for women's right to choose breast augmentation and has spoken before the FDA on several occasions in support of that right.

Procedures: Breast augmentation; Age: 31; Marital status: Married

(Stories contributed by NICOLE appear in Chapters 3, 6, 7, 9, 10 and Appendix 9: Additional stories for. Chapters 7, 9 and 10.)

Norma Jean is a Cosmetic Surgery Questionnaire Respondent who selected the following descriptors of herself: *family and relationship oriented, career oriented, outgoing and extraverted, liberal values and thoughts, innovative and creative* and *intellectual*. Not surprising for someone with such great self-esteem, on a scale of 1 to 5 (with 5 being the highest), she rated her attractiveness as 5.

Procedures: Nose: Age 36; lower facelift: Age: 44; Marital status: Married

(Stories contributed by NORMA JEAN appear in Chapters 1, 7, 10 and Appendix 9: Additional stories for Chapters 1 and 10.)

Pamela
Procedures: Facelift, eyes, neck, nose; Age: 53; Marital status: Single

(Stories about PAMELA that appear in Chapters 4 and 7 were contributed by Denise Thomas.)

Paula was a preschool teacher for eight years before she and her partner uprooted themselves from their comfortable lifestyle to become Peace Corp volunteers. Stationed in Romania, they assisted with Community Economic Development projects related to farm management and agribusiness. Paula said that although the work was hard and the comforts *nearly nonexistent*, the rewards were immeasurable. Once she and her partner returned to the United States, they opened a Bed and Breakfast Inn and Holistic Center in western Massachusetts.
Procedures: Facelift, eyes; Age: 43; Marital status: Partner relationship
(A story contributed by PAULA appears in Chapter 9.)

Peggy is a crime scene investigator who appeared on a TV episode of *Extreme Makeover*.
Procedures: Facelift, eyes; Age: 46; Marital status: Divorced
(A story about PEGGY appears in Chapter 1.)

'Realtor' is a Questionnaire Respondent, who listed *Don't want others to regard me as vain or shallow* as her main reason for not telling too many people about her surgery. Although happy with the results, she did not feel that she experienced any lifestyle or psychological impacts and took her surgery *pretty much in stride.* When asked to rate the factors that contribute to her feelings of positive self-image, she selected: *Love from another person* and *Confidence in my abilities* as the top two criteria with *My physical appearance* much further down on the list. **'Realtor'**, holds both undergraduate and post-graduate degrees. She has special interests in art, golf and travel.
Procedures: Facelift, eyes; Age: 64; Marital status: Married
(Stories contributed by REALTOR appear in Chapters 6 and 10.)

Ricki
(The story about RICKI that appears in Chapter 8 was contributed by Dorothy Birnham.)

Rita Spina, one of the women I interviewed who never had any cosmetic surgery, explains the reasons for her ambivalences in Chapter 8: *What Deters Us?,* where her full profile is embedded into the text. Rita's compassion and perceptiveness have touched my life in several compelling ways.
(**The story about RITA that appears in Chapter 8 was the result of a lengthy telephone interview and several e-mail messages between the two of us.**)

Rochelle had sent a letter to Newsday seeking advice about a facelift. I responded and we spoke on the phone. I don't know if she ever pursued it further. If she reads this profile, I hope she contacts me!
(**A story about ROCHELLE appears in Chapter 9.**)

Rose is a clinical psychologist with an active private practice. She is also the mother of a teenage daughter whom she says *constantly challenges my skills*. She is a regular at her local gym and competes in body building competitions. Although born and raised in New York State, **Rose** is bilingual, speaking Italian almost as fluently as English.
Procedures: Nose; Age: 37; Marital status: Divorced
(**Stories contributed by Rose appear in Chapters 3, 4, 7, 9 and Appendix 9: Additional stories for Chapter 6.**)

Rosalie Cropper was my first shift private duty nurse, who literally *weathered the storms* to get to my house on that immediate post surgery evening and was a great help and comfort during those first hours of recovery.
(**Stories about ROSALIE appear in Chapter 10 and the Epilogue.**)

Sara
Procedures: Facelift, eyes; Age: 68; Marital status: Married
(**The story about SARA that appears in Chapter 1 was contributed by Dorothy Birnham.**)

'Small' is a Questionnaire Respondent who said that she had *extremely low self-esteem* and was *quite self-conscious about* *specific body features* prior to surgery. She was motivated to do something to reverse those feelings after *looking at so many beautiful women all the time and wanting their bodies.* She does not feel that cosmetic surgery has changed any of her basic feelings about herself and is considering undergoing further cosmetic procedures.

Procedures: Tummy tuck, liposuction; Age: 33; Marital status: Single (A story contributed by 'SMALL' appears in Chapter 6.)

'Snowbird' is a Questionnaire Respondent who stated that she healed more slowly than she had anticipated. On a 1-5 rating scale, (with 1 being the lowest and 5 the highest), she selected 4 as her level of satisfaction with her ultimate surgical results, and says that she feels *younger and more energetic* since her facelift, *but also somewhat self-indulgent.* She indicated minimal emotional impacts to her surgery. **'Snowbird'** describes herself as *family and relationship oriented,* with *traditional values and thoughts.* Golf and Bridge are two of her favorite leisure time pursuits. She is both a mother and grandmother.

Procedures: Facelift, eyes; Age: 66; Marital status: Married (A story contributed by SNOWBIRD appears in Chapters 6.)

Stacey Lanza was my second shift private duty nurse during that first post surgery evening. She had to travel some distance to be with me during that strong Feb. blizzard, but I am glad she made that extra effort. I was ready for a little humor and found her stories so entertaining, her care, so comforting.

(Stories contributed by STACEY appear in Chapters 10 and the Epilogue.)

Stanley is a plastic surgeon whom I met by chance several months after my surgery. His candid assessment of my surgical results is detailed in the Epilogue of this book.

'Sunshine' is a Questionnaire Respondent who said that she had become somewhat self-conscious about the appearance of her neck because *I looked like a chicken.* On a scale of 1 to 10 (with 10 being the highest rating), she is the only respondent who listed her pre-surgery happiness level as 10. Although she now feels *prettier and more self-confident*, she does not believe that cosmetic surgery had any particular impact on her self-esteem. Sunshine is an attorney living in Scottsdale, Arizona.

Procedures: Neck: Age: 62; Nose: Age 18; Marital status: Married

(Stories contributed by SUNSHINE appear in Chapters 6 and 10.)

Susanne S. Warfield is President/CEO of Paramedical Consultants, Inc. and their publishing division, which publishes PCI Journal™, the official journal of the Society of Dermatology SkinCare Specialists. She is the leading expert on the business, legal and liability issues that affect physician and esthetician relationships and has authored or co-authored eight textbooks for the industry, including: *Legal & Liability Issues of a Medical Spa* and *Estheticians Guide to Working with Physicians.* Susanne serves as the Executive Director of both the National Coalition of Estheticians, Manufacturers/Distributors & Associations and the Society of Dermatology SkinCare Specialists. On a personal note, she is an avid rollerblader and diver. who recently completed her Divemaster Certification with future plans to become a Dive Instructor. Her other leisure time pursuits include pampering her "two wonderful dogs", hiking and gardening at her home in Ridgewood, NJ.

Sydney, a realtor working for a large residential real estate company, says she has done quite well for herself because of a decade long boom in home sales. She is a single mother of one grown son. An expert bridge player, **Sydney** once gave bridge lessons to the passengers on a cruise ship headed for the Bahamas in exchange for her free passage.

Procedures: Facelift, eyes, neck, brow lift; Age: 60; Marital status: Divorced

(A story contributed by SYDNEY appears in Chapter 7.)

Tanya
Procedures: Breast lift; Age: 38; Marital status: Married
(Stories about **Tanya**, that appear in Chapters 1 and Chapter 3, were contributed by Denise Thomas.)

Teresa is a psychiatric social worker whom I have known since early childhood. Living in a large suburban Long Island community, she has an active home office practice, but also finds time for her favorite hobbies of folk dancing and vegetarian cooking.
(Stories contributed by TERESA appear in Chapters 11 and 12.)

Tina is an art teacher living in San Diego, California. She has channeled her artistic flair into creating miniature porcelain dolls, complete with human hair and clothing representative of their individual nations. The production of these dolls began as a hobby, but evolved into a part time business. **Tina's** husband photographs each doll and has built her an Internet presence from which they are displayed and sold. She and her husband own a thirty foot sailboat and spend frequent weekends afloat.
Procedures: Breast lift; Age: 51; Marital status: Married
(A story contributed by TINA appears in Chapter 7.)

Val is a hairstylist with a devoted clientele who have been known to follow her as she moves on from one salon to the next. Not only does she know how to handle hair, but she has a great personality - an interesting conversationalist, perceptive and intelligent, with a cute sense of humor. A single mother since age twenty-one, **Val** has a beautiful face and figure to match, which totally belie her age, as she looks more teenage than middle age. A former jazz dance instructor, ardent Yoga enthusiast and proud owner of a Harley motorcycle; this soft spoken gal frequently hops on that Harley and takes off for a weekend trip with some of her friends.
Procedures: Facelift, eyes; Age: 54; Marital status: Divorced
(Stories contributed by VAL appear in Chapters 1, 9, 10 and 12.)

Vivian is another good friend whom I designated a member of my experimental group. *(See Appendix 9 for an explanation of this fun experiment.)* I call Vivian my walking encyclopedia friend. She has such knowledge of history and art that every outing with her - be it to a museum, art gallery or the streets of New York - is like being accompanied by your personal tour guide.

(Stories contributed by VIVIAN appear in Chapters 3, 9 and Appendix 9: Additional stories for my Epilogue.)

Whitney was born and raised in the suburbs of Cincinnati, Ohio, and remained there until retirement. For a number of years, she and her husband wintered in Scottsdale Arizona, where she continued to enjoy her favorite hobbies of golf, quilting, needlepoint and antiquing; but they have recently relocated to the West Coast of Florida. Whitney is an attractive blond who is full of bubbling energy, an outgoing personality and ready smile. The mother of three grown children, her daughter, Kelley, tells me she has *an incredible number of friends*. Whitney and I share something very special in common - our granddaughter, Emily! It was during a family reunion/vacation in Florida that I interviewed **Whitney** on the beaches of Siesta Key.

Procedures: Upper and lower eye lifts, laser resurfacing; Age: 63; Marital status: Married

(Stories contributed by WHITNEY appear in Chapters 7 and 9.)

Winnie is a retired social worker who raised her three children near the bay area in a woodsy suburban community of Suffolk County, NY. A former runner, she now settles for a slightly slower pace with active daily outdoor walks, weather permitting, and the use of her treadmill on days of inclement weather. She describes herself as "a people person and a good partner for my husband", but she also finds time to pursue some of her special interests of gardening, quilting and sewing. She and her husband are grandparents to seven grandchildren.

Procedures: Breast reduction; Age: 56; Full facelift, eyes, chin implant; Age: 60; Marital status: Married
(A story contributed by WINNIE appears in Chapter 9.)

Zena, a former fashion model, is now a successful journalist who writes freelance articles for women's magazines. She has a special talent for accessorizing clothing. You can count on Zena to know just how to wrap a shawl around her tall, slim frame to best advantage or how to select just the right piece of jewelry to transform an unremarkable outfit into a grand statement. This mother of twin girls is a gourmet cook. For her next project, she is considering creating a cookbook filled with favorite recipes that have been photographed on elegantly set tables.
Procedures: Facelift, eyes, neck; Age: 48; Marital status: Married
(Stories contributed by ZENA appear in Chapters 4, 6 and 9.)

Appendix 9 - Additional Stories

Gina's Story: "One evening my husband suddenly looked up and said: 'I don't think you even realize this about yourself, but you have become a much more sexual person since your cosmetic surgery. You can be busy with a million things, but if something sex related comes on the screen or into someone else's conversation, suddenly you perk up and give it your full attention.' I was somewhat aware of this, but he laid it out in the open for me." (**Gina** was shy about revealing details that might identify herself and preferred to remain completely anonymous).

(Stories contributed by Gina appear in Chapters 1, 3 and 4 and in Appendix 9: Additional stories for Chapter 1.)

Jody subtly alluded to her heightened sexuality after her cosmetic surgery when she said: *Denise, let me tell you, Victoria's Secret never looked so good!*

Procedures: Tummy tuck and Liposuction; Age: 26; Marital status: Single

(Stories about JODY which appear in Chapter 1 and in Appendix 9: Additional stories for Chapter 1 were contributed by Denise Thomas.)

Kelly: "I had breast augmentation and an eye lift. It's made me feel sexier. I walk around with a smile on my face most of the day. And yes, it has improved my sex life."

(Stories contributed by KELLY appear in Chapter 3 and in Appendix 9: Additional stories for Chapter 1.)

Norma Jean, a woman who responded to my Cosmetic Surgery Questionnaire, indicated that she was thirty-six when she had a rhinoplasty and at age forty-four had a lower facelift. You will read about her experiences with these surgeries in Chapter 10, *Misperceptions and Misconceptions* and her motivations for each one in Chapter 7, *What Propels Us*. I include her here because I just loved this gal's fantastic self-esteem! She responded to my questionnaire with a rating of *Extremely attractive* for her appearance both before and after her surgeries and felt that others would rate her similarly. As for sex, she wrote in all caps:
"I ALWAYS LOVED SEX BEFORE AND STILL LOVE IT NOW."
(Stories contributed by NORMA JEAN appear in Chapters 7, 10 and in Appendix 9: Additional stories for Chapters 1 and 10.)

Hope, a Floridian 'Snowbird' and cosmetic surgery questionnaire respondent summed up her feelings succinctly with her checked off responses: "I radiate more energy and zest for living. "I'm happier, more content." and "I take more interest in myself now." She further indicated that she now exercises regularly and takes better care of her skin. Before her facelift, on a scale of 1 to 10 (with 1 being the lowest and 10 the highest) she rated her pre-surgery happiness level a 6, and her post surgery happiness level an 8.5.
(Stories contributed by HOPE appear in Chapter 6, 10 and Appendix 9: Additional stories for Chapter 3.)

Lois: "Many women talked about changing their hair. I can identify. After wearing my hair shortly cropped and ash brown for over twenty years, I have become an experimenter of different hairstyles and colors. **Diane** and **Anne** both spoke about changing their hair color after cosmetic surgery and how good they felt when others noticed and complimented them about their new highlights."

Gail: "Okay, here goes. I had this one fantasy thing that I kept replaying in my head. I am in a beautiful mansion with a huge dance floor. It was a fairly formal affair attended by my plastic surgeon, his friends and office staff. Everyone knew that this was the night he was going to introduce his new love, but no one knew who she was, except he and me. He walks around the room greeting all his guests. I'm way off in the corner of the room, laughing and talking with a few people. We can hear soft music coming from the piano, then violins. A singer croons: "Baby, baby, I would never fall in love with one sweeter than you." He works his way toward me and smiles. I break free of the group I am with and take several steps in his direction. He reaches out to me and as we swirl across the floor, the guests beam and applaud. The vocalist continues: "I would never find another love as precious as you . . ." By now my arms are around his neck, fingers interlocked behind his head, as we stare into each other's eyes and I sing softly into his ear. I never let myself think in terms of what happened later in the evening. The romance part was more exciting than sex."
(Stories contributed by GAIL appear in Chapters 1, 3, 6, 12 and Appendix 9: Additional stories for Chapter 6.)

Judy: "I understand what you are saying because I was even drawn to my breast surgeon, Dr. Virginia Mauer, who is a woman. I found her sense of confidence and self-esteem so appealing, like a mother with her child. I still think she is the most incredible woman. She even established the Mauer Foundation for Breast Health Education, which is a public educational resource to promote breast health.**(Stories contributed by JUDY appear in Chapters 1, 3, 6 and Appendix 9: Additional stories for Chapter 6.)**

Julie: "My husband died after a massive heart attack during a tennis match. He was only thirty-six years old. It was so sudden. Here I was, a widow with two small children living on the West Coast apart from family and most of my friends. I was devastated, overwhelmed, beyond sad. I went through the motions of living, but I felt dead inside.

After awhile my eyes looked like slits, probably from all the crying I had done. My friend suggested that I go to her plastic surgeon and have my eyes done. She thought it would give me a lift. I agreed that it might be a good idea, a way to make me feel a little more upbeat. When I went for a consultation, he gave me lots of compliments about my appearance. I felt flattered and immediately scheduled my surgery. It came out okay and it did make me feel better about myself, but at a huge price." (See Chapter 6 for the remainder of Julie's story.)

(The stories contributed by Julie appear in Chapter 6 and Appendix 9: Additional stories for Chapter 6.)

Rose: "About two years after my surgery, I was in an auto accident and had to go to the emergency room. I asked for the plastic surgeon who had done my nose because I liked his work, and to be quite honest, I was already attracted to him. As he stitched up the laceration on my chin, we spoke about our current marital situations. (We were both recently separated from our spouses.) Before our conversation was over, he had invited me out for dinner. We had such fun together. He had a really good sense of humor and made me laugh so much. He used to joke about the letters MD – that they really stood for Major Deity! Then we began to date rather seriously, a fact that will become obvious when I tell you this next part. As our relationship developed, I couldn't help but notice how comfortable he was with a woman's body. That was a very special part of our relationship. So yes, to answer your question, I did feel physically attracted to him."

(Stories contributed by ROSE appear in Chapters 3, 4, 7 and 9 and Appendix 9: Additional stories for Chapter 6.)

Anne: ". . . I knew I would never look twenty-one again. That wasn't my goal. I just didn't want to look like a worn fifty-five. I knew that the best creams, lotions and make-up wouldn't change it. Exercise and diet wouldn't change it. Only surgery would do the trick. Getting back to your question of enhancing sexuality as a reason for undergoing cosmetic surgery, I would say it was definitely part of the package."
(Stories contributed by ANNE appear in Chapters 1, 3, 7, 9 and 10 and Appendix 9: Additional stories for Chapter 7.)

Barbara: "I went for cosmetic surgery because no amount of diet or exercise would slim my legs, but liposuction of my legs and thighs did the trick."
(Stories contributed by BARBARA appear in Chapter 9 and Appendix 9: Additional stories for Chapters 7 and 10.)

Donna: "Oh, my, how do I even begin to say this to you? This is so very private, but you're such an accepting person that I feel I can share this with you. About a year before my surgery, I went through a kind of mid-life crisis. I became involved in an adult chat room, and it really opened my eyes in a kind of playful way. . . . I would say that this chat room was responsible for helping me grow and explore in ways I never had done before. I have a very busy practice, but somehow this became a priority in my life and I found the time. I might add, I'm not even a baby boomer. As a matter of fact, I'm nearing that big 6 - 0 birthday. I had a very strict upbringing, so I never allowed this type exploration to be part of my thinking before. Now that I'm talking to you, it's all coming together for me. I really think there is a connection between my personal sexual awakening and my desire for cosmetic surgery."

(Stories contributed by DONNA appear in Chapter 7 and Appendix 9: Additional stories for Chapter 7.)

Judith: "I couldn't stand looking in the mirror any more. It was my jowls more than anything that bothered me, but I had a total facelift, lower eyes, neck and forehead done. I used a plastic surgeon who runs a clinic in Florida. His patients come to his Manhattan office for their consultations, but then go to Florida for their surgery. After surgery you recuperate in his clinic for one week where you are pampered and given total care, including all meals, just like at a fine spa. By the time I came home, I already looked great. The results were so natural. I met some new friends at the clinic. We still meet for periodic reunions and playfully call ourselves *The New Faces Club*."

(Stories contributed by JUDITH appear in Chapter 7 and Appendix 9: Additional stories for Chapters 7 and 9.)

Lauren: "I've never really focused on age because I've always looked young and felt the way I looked. However, over the last few years I'd noticed subtle changes in my jaw line and neck that only hinted at what was to come. One day when I was in a store holding up chandelier earrings to see the effect, I noticed how they accentuated my jaw line. It made me feel old to see this and was especially discouraging since I feel so young and my body still looks as young as I feel. I decided to proceed with cosmetic surgery before these changes were so apparent to other people and before the older appearance got me down. My mother, who is in her eighties, still looks unbelievably young except for her very sagging neck. I knew that would be my future if I didn't have some surgery so I decided to take things into my own hands and turn back the clock. By the way, my mother still laments the fact that she never did anything about her neck."

(Stories contributed by LAUREN appear in Chapters 1, 7, 9, 10 and Appendix 9: Additional stories for Chapters 7 and 10.)

Nancy: "I knew I might lose sensation in my breasts, but I didn't even care because I wanted to have smaller breasts. Not only was I self-conscious about their size, but it was hard to get clothes that fit right. I had to get many of my clothes tailored – either enlarged on top or taken in on the bottom. If I bought separates, I would always get a bigger size for the top half of me."

(Stories contributed by NANCY appear in Chapter 3 and Appendix 9: Additional stories for Chapter 7).

Nicole: "When I was twelve years old, I had a benign breast tumor. After it was removed, that breast was less full and smaller than the other breast. . . . I didn't even know about breast augmentation then, didn't know this could be an option for me. I had an older cousin who was very flat chested. She had breast augmentation and when she showed me her results, I thought her breasts were just beautiful. But I still wasn't thinking much about that for myself. . . . But when I stopped nursing, my breasts looked worse than prior to pregnancy. Whereas before I was small, I was still perky and firm. I could live with that. During my second pregnancy, I began to research breast augmentation surgery."

(Stories contributed by NICOLE appear in Chapter 1, 3, 6, 7, 9, 10, and Appendix 9: Additional stories for Chapters 7, 9 and 10.)

Jane: "I asked several women I know who have had cosmetic surgery if they would be willing to answer your questionnaire. None of them wanted to do it. They all gave excuses: "I'm really too busy.", "I'm having company next week.", things like that. I stressed that it was completely anonymous but that didn't seem to help. I just think it makes a lot of people uncomfortable to have to think about their feelings. They had the surgery and that's over with. They would rather not deal with those feelings, because it makes them uncomfortable on some level."

(Stories contributed by JANE appear in Chapters 7, 9, 10. and Appendix 9: Additional stories for Chapters 9 and 10.)

Judith: "People are much more open now about cosmetic surgery. It's like looking on the Internet for a date. Years ago very few people did that, but today it's commonplace and an accepted means of meeting people. People are more open in their sexuality too. We just live with much less secrecy in our lives."

(Stories contributed by JUDITH appear in Chapter 9 and Appendix 9: Additional stories for Chapters 7 and 9.)

Lois: Story 1

I told both my daughters-in-law about my impending surgery. The next day I got phone calls from both of my sons. With typical male reserve, each one waited for me to bring up the subject. Larry asked lots of questions. The chin implant got a real rise out of him. *Mom, I never even knew they did that!* When I asked David for his reaction, he said, *Look, Mom, if it's going to make you feel better, go for it.* I was grateful neither of them tried to dissuade me.

Lois: Story 2
"The week before my surgery I had lunch with my friend **Bobbi**, so she automatically became a member of my control group. Bobbi looked at me with an expression that spoke louder than words. 'Lois, of all my friends, you are the one I would have thought least likely to go for a facelift', she finally chuckled."

Lois: Story 3: "After my surgery, I wanted to tell my friend **Joan**, but somehow couldn't get up the courage. Joan is somewhat older than I - just old enough to have absorbed some of those really negative attitudes about cosmetic surgery that were once so prevalent. She's a person you can count on to tell you just what she's thinking, and although I generally enjoy her candor, I was afraid I'd get some negative vibes here.'

"At the end of one phone conversation I finally broached the subject. 'Joan there is something I've been wanting to talk to you about, but I just haven't had the courage', I say. 'Oh, dear, what did I do now?' she asks. I told her that it was nothing she did, but that before she learned this from someone else, I wanted to tell her that I had had a facelift. She told me that she had been looking at me at a friend's house that prior week, thinking how great I looked and even commented to her husband: 'I know Lois changed her hairstyle, but she looks so pretty. Could hair make such a difference?' She was more intrigued than anything else. She asked me lots of questions; but when I didn't detect any value judgment, I relaxed a bit more."

Lois: Story 4

"I was particularly concerned about telling **Lee**, a delightfully refreshing member of our book group, who wears no make-up to enhance her pretty face or twinkling eyes, no hair color to conceal the increasing strands of gray in her hair. A horticulturist by profession, she enjoys nothing more than digging her hands into fresh soil. Lee was puzzled as to why I would be particularly concerned about her. 'But you're so natural', I explained. 'I just didn't think it was something that would appeal to you.' 'But you see, I love aesthetics', was her spontaneous response."

Marilyn: "It took a couple of weeks before I wanted to be seen by anyone, but now, almost four months later, I know I look so much younger and am thrilled with the results. My new colleagues treat me like I am much younger than my actual age, giving me advice about steps to take to assure myself of getting tenure, never suspecting that I am near retirement."

(Stories contributed by MARILYN appear in Chapters 7, 9 and 10. and Appendix 9: Additional stories for Chapters 9 and 10.)

Nicole: "I only told my sister, my parents and my best friend. I just knew what reaction I'd get and I didn't want to deal with that. Women are a little more open about breast augmentation today, but still most are secretive. Women who do research on my website still tell me they don't want people talking about them. In my own situation, I hadn't told my sister-in-law or her husband anything about my plans to have this surgery. Afterwards I dressed in overall shorts and a T-shirt the first time I was going to see them. I wrongly believed that the bib of the overalls would sort of hide everything. But they took one look at me and said: "What did you do to yourself?" So I told them. They were quite upset that I had kept it a secret and that I did not think to confide in them, but in the end they understood."

(Stories contributed by NICOLE appear in Chapters 1, 3, 6, 7, 9 and 10 and Appendix 9: Additional stories for Chapters 7, 9, and 10.)

Anne: "I understood most of the process before hand. It wasn't any deep mystery to me. Once I felt comfortable with my surgeon and the facility, I was fine about the surgery. The night before my surgery, I visited my daughter, who helped keep me busy by shopping with her for little gifts to bring back to family members."
(Stories contributed by ANNE appear in Chapters 1, 3, 7, 9, 10 and in Appendix 9: Additional stories for Chapters 7 and 10.)

Diane: "The night before my surgery I was very nervous and when I get nervous, my whole body shakes. But strangely, the next day I felt calm yet energized. I was so focused on the fact that I would look better and was excited to see the outcome. I had such confidence in my surgeon."
(Stories contributed by DIANE appear in Chapters 3, 7, 9 and Appendix 9: Additional stories for Chapter 10.)

Denise Thomas: "I ease the way for many of my pre-surgery clients by introducing them to some of my clients who have already undergone similar procedures with the same surgeon and are willing to share their experiences. I believe this makes a real difference in their comfort level. I tell my clients they should be thrilled that they are doing such a wonderful thing for themselves. Then I give them the following advice:

> "Trust your doctor. He has already proven himself to be one of the best. Don't start giving him cautions about doing too much of this or too little of that. Let him do his work. You just relax and enjoy it. Focus on the new you and how happy you will be."

Denise tells why she prefers solo practitioners to those with some sort of partnership arrangement.

> "Although I know that some very competent surgeons work with partners or associates, I only recommend solo practitioners. I believe a solo practice speaks to the success of the physician because he has no need to share office expenses to make his practice financially viable. Furthermore, I believe that when a patient goes to a solo practitioner, she is likely to receive more personalized attention from the entire office staff."

Hewitt: "I was jittery, but that's just my nature. I think people often don't ask their friends and just imagine the worst."
(Stories contributed by HEWITT appear in Chapter 7 and Appendix 9: Additional stories for Chapter 10.)

Jane: "Although I have always been nervous prior to going to the dentist, for a physical examination or especially for any type of surgery; I was not at all nervous before my cosmetic surgery. I was excited and energized by the thought of a better me. My husband had always been opposed to any type of cosmetic surgery because he had viewed many poor results where women were left with artificial faces devoid of expression. About two months before surgery, when I told him my decision, he was not happy but could not convince me to change my mind. A week before surgery I decided that I would NOT let my husband drive me to the doctor's office, although he did offer. Instead I hired a limo to take me there and a nurse to escort me home and remain with me for the next twenty-four hours. I could not believe that fear or nervousness never entered my mind. I was completely focused on becoming a better me."
(Stories contributed by JANE appear in Chapters 7, 9, 10 and Appendix 9: Additional stories for Chapters 9 and 10.)

Lauren: "When I arrived in the city two days before my surgery I was a basket case. The reality of what I was about to do finally hit. However, the day before my surgery, my daughter kept me busy shopping and the distraction was just what I needed. My doctor instructed me to take a Dramamine one hour before the surgery. I was amazingly calm the morning of the surgery anyway, but I'm sure the Dramamine helped. I was the first procedure of the day so I didn't have to wait and stress. Unfortunately there were many mirrors in my hotel suite where I recovered so it was hard to avoid seeing my reflection.

(Stories contributed by LAUREN appear in Chapters 1, 7, 9, 10 and Appendix 9: Additional stories for Chapters 7 and 10.)

Maria: "I went to a wedding the night before surgery. It helped so much to be around other people. I had a wonderful friend who was with me that night and took me to my surgeon the next morning."

(Stories contributed by MARIA appear in Chapter 10 and Appendix 9: Additional stories for Chapter 10.)

Marilyn: "On the day of surgery, I was driving my car up Third Avenue when I said to my husband sitting beside me: 'I need to turn around and go home. I just can't go through with this.' But somehow I kept going and as soon as we arrived at the doctor's office, I was given a pill to relax me. Then I was fine. I was starting a new job two months after my surgery and one of my biggest fears was that I wouldn't be all healed before I came face to face with all these new people."

(Stories contributed by MARILYN appear in Chapters 9, 10 and Appendix 9: Additional stories for Chapters 9 and 10.)

Nicole - Story 1: "I agonized forever until I made the decision to go for surgery. The day of surgery I kept saying: 'I must be out of my mind. I have two little children. What if I die?' I also felt guilt over spending so much money on this."

Nicole – Story 2: "Women seem to go through two stages. At first they are most concerned about pain and spending so much money on themselves. Some feel they are not worth it. Then once they make the decision to go ahead with surgery, they begin to focus on other concerns like anesthesia, complications, what size breasts to choose. They will talk to me about concerns they feel embarrassed to discuss with their doctors. For example, they worry about loss of nipple sensation after surgery. I tell women that it is important for them to talk to their doctors about these concerns.

"You need to take control. He can't read your mind."
(Stories contributed by NICOLE appear in Chapters 1, 3, 6, 7, 9, 10, Appendix 9: Additional stories for Chapters 7, 9, and 10.)

🔖 **Note:** As the creator and owner of the largest Internet resource for breast augmentation and the leader of support groups, Nicole has had vast experiences with women and breast augmentation issues.

Norma Jean - Story 1: "I was high for the seven days I was on painkillers and laughed each time I saw what could have been a huge mistake. One week later, when my bandages were removed, I remember staring at the mirror and crying from relief because I looked just like me, only better. Eight years later I still love my nose and think the best part of all is that it will never grow again."
(Stories contributed by NORMA JEAN appear in Chapter 7, 10 and Appendix 9: Additional stories for Chapters 1 and 10.)

Norma Jean – Story 2: "I was fine until I entered my room in the hospital and changed into a hospital gown. I got so scared that I nearly bolted from the room. I remember crying out for valium. Then I was calm.
(Stories contributed by NORMA JEAN appear in Chapters 7, 10 and Appendix 9: Additional stories for Chapters 1 and 10.)

Lois: Once my surgery was scheduled, I decided to conduct a little experiment. I would tell three friends in advance, *my control group*, and select three others to whom I would give no advance notice, *my experimental group*. My criteria for selection was based solely on this single factor: those I saw closest to my surgery date would be the controls, simply because I knew that during those last few days I would be bursting to talk and it would be the most difficulty time for me to guard my secret. (When I gave Ken an early draft of my manuscript to read, and he got to this section, he wrote in the margin: "That's you. Most would remain mute. And you can quote me here.") I also knew that my controls, those who knew in advance, would be programmed to say I looked great. After all, that's what friends are for. But would those without foreknowledge notice changes to my appearance? It was a fun experiment that I recommend to others.

Evelyn was one of my 'experimental group' friends who saw me about ten days post surgery, before I was entirely healed. We attended a wake together, but while enroute, she was focused on her driving, and didn't comment on my appearance. But when we finally came face to face inside the funeral home, the game began with her first comment: "Your eyes look nice." Then she looked some more and said, "How did you get that bruise on your cheek?" I said something stupid, like: "I think I bumped into something. I'm not really sure." I see that she keeps staring, trying to make sense of what she sees. "Something is different. Your look great. What is it?" I didn't want to start a whole discussion inside the funeral home, so I just say, "Evelyn, take a good look", as I roll down my cowl neck blouse to reveal my bruises. She nearly exploded with surprise. "Oh, my God, I can't believe it. When?" Back in her kitchen several hours later, she asked for the details. As we spoke, her enthusiasm grew. "The thing is, it's so natural. No one would ever look at you and say you had a facelift. One of my colleagues had cosmetic surgery, but her face is so tight, you can almost guess it at a glance. Wow! You just look wonderful! What an exciting couple of weeks. Let's see – what exciting news do I have for you? The only thing I did this past two weeks was have a colonoscopy."

That Saturday evening we attended a concert with Evelyn and Sam. I sat opposite Sam during dinner. "Don't be insulted", Evelyn whispers. "Sam doesn't notice these things." He didn't. I wasn't.

About three weeks after surgery, I met Vivian, another experimental group member, for breakfast. We talked about books for a while, but I noticed that she kept looking at me quizzically. Then suddenly she blurted out, "Lois, you did your eyes." As she continued to look some more, I noticed her touching the lower portion of her own face. "Something else", she finally said. "Lois, I don't believe it. You look fabulous. That's it. I'm doing it!" But she never did.

The reactions from casual observers varied from amusing, to exhilarating. Here are a few I recall: I went to a retiree luncheon where the president of the association greeted me with a near shriek as she blurted out: "Your hair looks smashing." On my first day back on the tennis courts, one of my partners gushed, "Your make-up looks fantastic!" I was asked for proof of age when I extended my senior citizen train ticket to the conductor on the LIRR. A member of my investment club did a double take when I arrived and said:

"You look great. Have you been on vacation?" Let's face it. We all like looking good, getting compliments, even though it isn't our raison d'etre. I admit it. I am no exception. That recognition felt good.

But I also felt 'attitude' and veiled criticism from others. Negative attitudes are not often voiced, but nonetheless can be sensed. It is best to stay clear of all forms of negativity, especially immediately before and after surgery.

CR

The central messages of *Sex, Lies and Cosmetic Surgery* are only beginning to emerge beyond the confines of this book. Based on a study of 70 women who completed a survey about their postoperative psychosexual life, the ASAPS posted the following headline at their website: www.surgery.org/ as this book was about to go to press:

"Women's Self-Image and Sexual Satisfaction Increase After Cosmetic Surgery"

It is gratifying to learn that the validity of the work I began in Feb. 2001 continues to be confirmed.

If you have a story to share, please visit my website at www.sexliesandcosmeticsurgery.com where we can meet and chat. I will continue to post your stories online and look forward to speaking with you.

My very best,

Lois

Lois W. Stern

Sex, Lies and Cosmetic Surgery CD

You can order this CD with its ten different self-assessment quizzes, evaluation forms and checklists at: www.sexliesandcosmeticsurgery.com/

(Email cosmeticsurgery@optonline.net to request pricing information for bulk orders of 10 or more CD's or books.)

Or complete the cut-out order form below, enclose a check made payable to *Personalized Stories, Inc.* and mail the order form along with your check to:

Personalized Stories
CD Offer
c/o Box 2229
Huntington, NY 11743

Sex, Lies and Cosmetic Surgery CD
Regularly $18.95

Special offer with this coupon: $9.95 (Plus $3.75 for shipping/handling of one or two CD's sent to same address)

Please print clearly. This is your address label.

Name _____

Address _____

_____

_____

E-mail address _____

Phone _____
  (In case there is a question about your order)

❧ About the Author ☙

"When I was 4 ½ years old, I remember being sent to my room for a nap, but instead of resting, I practiced printing alphabet letters - all over my newly papered bedroom wall. What I most recall about that day was having to stand behind the dinette door, perched right next to my mother's old Singer Sewing Machine, until I apologized for my misbehavior. I couldn't understand why I was being punished for all my hard work, so I stood there for what seemed like hours, rather than say the simple words: *I'm sorry.* Fortunately this inauspicious beginning didn't dull my enthusiasm for writing."

During her twenty plus years as an educator, Lois W. Stern took an active role in her field as a frequent presenter at state and national educational conferences. Co-president of Suffolk Reading Council and subsequent Regional Director of Nassau and Suffolk LI Reading Councils, a number of her articles have been published by ERIC (U.S. Department of Education - Office of Educational Research and Improvement), parent newsletters, Newsday and the New York Times. As founder of Kidstories, Stern has authored children's books and poems that then become personalized with facts and photos of each child.

After retirement from education, Stern continued to pursue her love for writing, and soon became co-editor of a Long Island Internet web-zine, LI EYE. As she created and authored the column *Ordinary People, Extraordinary Lives,* she discovered her special niche of investigative journalism, and put those same talents to work in her book, ***Sex, Lies and Cosmetic Surgery***, where she was able to gain the trust of over 100 women while interviewing them about some of the most intimate aspects of their lives

Stern received a Bachelor of Science degree from Barnard College of Columbia University, where she majored in Sociology. She holds one Masters Degree in Elementary Education and a second in Reading and Special Education.